Embracing Special Needs Parenting With Wisdom
Find the Wisdom to Raise Your
Special Needs Child

By: Maria Cruz & Patrick Baldwin

Copyright 2018
American Christian Defense Alliance, Inc.
Baltimore, Maryland
ACDAInc.Org

All Rights Reserved. No part of this publication may be reproduced in any form or by any means, including scanning, photocopying, or otherwise without prior written permission of the copyright holder.

Special Request

Thank you for purchasing our book and supporting our Ministry. We actually have two requests – To Pray for Our Ministry and to Read this Book All the Way through. No Ministry can Survive without Prayers and Support so we ask you to keep our Ministry in Your Daily Prayers and Pray as the Lord leads.

We encourage you to Read the Book you purchased all the way through. Many Books NEVER Get Read, and the ones that do only get read the first few pages.

One of our Special Request is that if you are serious about learning the material in this book that you take time to actually read this book in its entirety – all the way through.

We all lead such busy lives nowadays and can get side tracked so easily, please take a moment to consider my words and read to the end of the book and keep us in Your Prayers.

Thank You once again for purchase. We deeply appreciate Your Prayers and Support and know that God will Bless You as You continue to Bless this Ministry.

Table of Contents

SPECIAL REQUEST 2

EMBRACING PREGNANCY, YOUR CHILD, AND PARENTING 7

CHAPTER 1: HANDLE WITH CARE 8

CHAPTER 2: THE MIRACLE OF LIFE 15

CHAPTER 3: MEANT TO BE PARENTS 20

CHAPTER 4: WE'RE HAVING A BABY 26

CHAPTER 5: THE FIRST TRIMESTER 34

CHAPTER 6: THE SECOND TRIMESTER 41

CHAPTER 7: THE THIRD TRIMESTER 47

CHAPTER 8: LET'S DO THIS 54

CHAPTER 9: FAMILY 59

CHAPTER 10: CHILDREN ARE THE FUTURE 63

PARENTING SPECIAL NEEDS CHILDREN 66

PRELUDE 67

CHAPTER 1: YOU ARE GOING TO BE THE PARENT OF A SPECIAL NEEDS CHILD 68

CHAPTER 2: GUARDING YOUR HEART, SOUL, MIND, AND STRENGTH 75

CHAPTER 3: TRUE LOVE IS DEVOID OF ALL PRIDE 98

CHAPTER 4: OVERCOMING THE EDUCATIONAL OBSTACLES 107

CHAPTER 5: WE ARE FAMILY 113

CHAPTER 6: LET YOUR "LIGHT" SHINE 118

CHAPTER 7: DEALING WITH SPECIAL SOCIAL AND COMMUNICATION NEEDS.......................................124

CHAPTER 8: DEALING WITH SPECIAL NEUROLOGICAL NEEDS 129

CHAPTER 9: DEALING WITH GENETIC AND PHYSICAL SPECIAL NEEDS..135

CHAPTER 10: YOUR NOT-SO-SECRET SECRET THOUGHTS 144

WISDOM FROM YOUR ELDERS 148

INTRODUCTION..149

CHAPTER 1: FOUNDATIONS OF RELATIONSHIPS 152

CHAPTER 2: BENEFITS FOR YOUNG PEOPLE 175

CHAPTER 3: BENEFITS FOR OLDER PEOPLE 183

CHAPTER 4: FOSTERING STRONG RELATIONSHIPS 188

CHAPTER 5: RELATIONSHIPS IN THE CHURCH 195

CHAPTER 6: A SENSE OF RESPONSIBILITY.................200

CHAPTER 7: PATIENCE 204

CHAPTER 8: FAITH 208

CHAPTER 9: UNCONDITIONAL LOVE 212

CHAPTER 10: WISDOM..217

SPECIAL GIFT	221
STAY IN CONTACT	223
FIND ALL OUR BOOKS	224
ADDITIONAL FORMATS	226

Embracing Pregnancy, Your Child, and Parenting

YOUR GUIDE BOOK TO LEARN HOW TO UNLOCK THE SECRETS OF SUCCESSFUL PARENTING

By: Maria Cruz & Patrick Baldwin

Chapter 1: Handle With Care

Psalm 127:3 says, *Children are a heritage from the Lord, offspring a reward from Him.*

...from the LORD—that's where our children come from. The LORD. He entrusts them to us to care for; helping them go from infancy to adulthood safely, securely, and in an atmosphere that reflects God's love as much as is humanly possible.

There are a number of verses and passages of scripture in the Bible that reflect and teach this truth. We'll be looking at several of them throughout the pages of this book. I want to begin, however, by taking a look into the heart and mind of the woman I consider to be the most Godly mother of all times. Her name: Hannah.

We are introduced to Hannah in the first chapter of the Old Testament book of First Samuel. Hannah, who is one of Elkanah's two wives, is a tender-hearted and Godly woman who desperately longs to be a mother.

Her inability to conceive a child is something Peninnah, Elkanah's other wife, takes great pleasure in. Peninnah's taunting and ridicule plants seeds of insecurity and doubt in Hannah's mind; doubts that Elkanah quickly puts to rest; assuring his sweet wife that his love for her is true—child or no child.

I'm sure this had to bring at least some degree of comfort to Hannah's heart and mind, but it didn't change the fact that Hannah wanted to be a mom more than anything in the world. Hannah knew, though, that wanting to be a mom wasn't enough. Hannah knew that the gift of motherhood came from one 'place' and one 'place' only—God.

So Hannah prayed. She prayed and she prayed and she prayed some more. But her prayers weren't 'just' to become a mom. Hannah told God that if He would bless her with a child she would give the child back to him—literally. She told God that if He would bless her with a son she would give him to Eli to be raised up as the next High Priest and Judge over all of Israel.

After praying the prayer Hannah and Elkanah conceived a child. When the baby was born they named him Samuel. And true to her word, when Samuel was about three or four years old Hannah took him to live in the Tabernacle with Eli so that he could learn the duties of the priesthood. Samuel grew up to be a man of deep faith and one who obeyed God to the letter. He was the last Judge of Israel before they demanded that He appoint someone to be their king.

I'm sharing Hannah's story with you to remind you that your children are on loan to you from God. You are their caretakers and their role models. God has charged you with the task, aka, given you the privilege of overseeing some of His most priceless treasures.

As a steward of these treasures you need to be sure you care for them the way God expects you to—the way He told us to in Deuteronomy 6:5-9:

And thou shalt love the Lord thy God with all thine heart, and with all thy soul, and with all thy might. And these words, which I command thee this day, shall be in thine heart: And thou shalt teach them diligently unto thy children, and shalt talk of them when thou sittest in thine house, and when thou walkest by the way, and when thou liest down, and when thou risest up. And thou shalt bind them for a sign upon thine hand, and they shall be as frontlets between thine eyes. And thou shalt write them upon the posts of thy house, and on thy gates.

You are to teach them diligently. When you teach diligently you teach consistently; meaning on a regular basis. But teaching with diligence also implies that you are meticulous and careful to make sure they don't just know *about* God, but that they know who God *is*—His character.

God doesn't just tell us the manner in which we are supposed to teach our children. No, God also gives us the specifics of how to get the job done. He tells us to **talk of them when thou sittest in thine house, and when thou walkest by the way.** He goes on to say we are to teach our children when they lay down and when they are awake. In other words, the Word of God is to permeate our children's lives. Their exposure to God's Word needs to be the norm—not the exception. We are to **teach our children to see God** in everything, **give thanks** to God for all things, **give God the credit** He is due, and **give God total control** of our lives.

And then He gets to the really personal part. Teaching our children these things needs to be done by example. Children really do learn what they live, and God is calling us to make sure they live in homes where God is first and foremost every day and in every way.

That's a pretty tall order—an awesome responsibility. It is not impossible, though, because God never gives you a job to do without also providing you with the resources necessary to do it...and do it well.

The Word of God ...prayer...the Holy Spirit...Godly counsel from other parents...a parent-heart that wants to give their children the best life possible—these are the resources we have at our disposal.

You need to know, however, that these resources aren't meant to be optional. Deuteronomy 6 isn't a suggestion or a wish. It is a command from the creator to the moms and dads He entrusts with His most priceless treasures.

Hannah knew she was raising Samuel *for* God. Raising your children *for* God is your job, too.

Chapter 2: The Miracle of Life

Have you ever looked at a newborn baby? I mean really looked—their tiny fingernails, the perfect little curvatures of their ears, the soft little eyelashes, the way they instinctively know when Mom is nearby? They are pure perfection, aren't they? They are also a living, breathing miracle.

Yes, life is a miracle. It couldn't just happen by accident. Too many things have to be just right in order for an egg and sperm to get together and stay that way. Oh, I know there are those first-time-I-had-sex-I-got-pregnant people out there. But they are far from the norm. In fact, the UK's Daily Mail website and the New York Post newspaper reported that research conducted on three thousand couples showed that on average, it takes couples one hundred and four sessions of lovemaking before pregnancy is achieved.

Additional research shows that less than half of all couples get pregnant within the first six months of trying to conceive, but that just over ninety percent conceive within a year. So like I said, there's nothing accidental or coincidental about it.

I also know that getting the news that you are expecting can take you on a rollercoaster of emotions. Excitement, disbelief, anxiousness, fear, awe, surprise, elation...and sometimes disappointment and anger are the most common.

Not every pregnancy is planned or desired. Most teenagers aren't trying to achieve pregnancy when they're in the back seat of a car or home alone on the couch. Sometimes couples don't feel ready to start a family for one reason or another, but find out they are anyway. Other couples feel their families are complete and/or are getting ready to be empty-nesters when suddenly….

For others—especially couples who have experienced the grief of miscarriage or infertility—pregnancies can be scary. They want it so badly they are too afraid to let themselves enjoy it. They don't want to get their hopes up only to have their hearts broken again.

And then there are those that count down the days from the time their chances of conceiving were the highest until they can take a pregnancy test to see if this will be the month.

No matter what you are feeling or thinking, though, you need to know that God knows exactly what's going on and he knows exactly what He is doing. He knew wayyyyyyyyy back when he said, "Let there be light…" when each of us would be conceived. I know that's a lot to wrap your head around, but it's true. The Bible says so in Psalm 139:15-16:

My frame was not hidden from You, When I was made in secret, And skillfully wrought in the lowest parts of the earth. Your eyes saw my substance, being yet unformed. And in Your book they all were written, The days fashioned for me, When as yet there were none of them. (NKJV)

Every mother out there can testify that giving birth and being a parent is truly a gift from God – The Miracle of Life if you would. Hopefully God will see fit in His plan to bless you abundantly with children in the near future. Just remember Children have angels assigned to watch over them so make sure you're gracious to strangers.

Hebrews 13:2 says, "Do not forget to show hospitality to strangers, for by so doing some people have shown hospitality to angels without knowing it."

As far as I know I've never welcomed an actual angel into my home, but I have been the recipient of their God-given ability to intervene in my life in a way that still leaves me 'on my knees thankful'.

Remember: Babies aren't made by accident. A mommy and daddy's perfect timing doesn't even guarantee anything. It is God's perfect timing that results in the miracle of life.

Chapter 3: Meant to be Parents

Genesis 1:27-28 says, "*So God created man in His own image; in the image of God He created him; male and female He created them. Then God blessed them, and God said to them, "Be fruitful and multiply; fill the earth and subdue it; have dominion over the fish of the sea, over the birds of the air, and over every living thing that moves on the earth."thing that moveth upon the earth."*

Genesis 9:1 says, "*So God blessed Noah and his sons, and said to them: "Be fruitful and multiply, and fill the earth."*

In Genesis 28:3, Isaac said to Jacob, "*May God Almighty bless you, And make you fruitful and multiply you, That you may be an assembly of peoples;*

And finally, Psalm 127:3-5 tells us, *"Lo, children are an heritage of the Lord: and the fruit of the womb is his reward. As arrows are in the hand of a mighty man; so are children of the youth. Happy is the man that hath his quiver full of them: they shall not be ashamed, but they shall speak with the enemies in the gate."*

It isn't difficult to see the common thread running through these four verses, is it?

God wants us to be parents. Next to worshipping Him and sharing the message of the Gospel to anyone and everyone we possibly can, being a parent is the most important job God gives us to do. Remember: the job of parent is synonymous with being the caretaker of God's most precious and priceless treasures…children.

Unfortunately, not every parent knows just how important their job is. If they did, the National Children's Alliance wouldn't have to report that over 700,000 children in the US are treated or receive some type of service because of abuse or neglect each and every year. Additionally, over 3 million children in this country are the subject of an intervention or protection order.

Why do you think this is? Why would anyone want to harm an innocent child? The answers to that question are varied. Some would say it is because the parents were abused or neglected, so they don't know any better. Others would say it is because these parents is not mature enough to be a parents. And still others would say that an abusive parent's actions are beyond their control because of an addiction or emotional/mental disorder. While these things may or may not be true, the real reason child abuse/neglect happen is because God is not present in the home. When God is absent from a home a lot of other things are absent, as well. Things like patience, gentleness, genuine selflessness, diligent teaching about God, and unconditional love.

As Christians we need to be conscientious about making sure God is present in our homes. We have the same perspective on parenting that God designed us to have. We need to make sure we embrace our role as parents; viewing it as a praiseworthy responsibility rather than a chore. It is a praiseworthy responsibility we need to take to heart.

Some would ask then, if being a parent is something God desires us to do, then why are there Christian couples suffering from infertility? And if being fruitful and multiplying is so important, then where does that leave couples who don't want children or those who don't marry? Are they living outside of God's will for mankind?

Infertility is an emotionally and physically painful condition. But know this…infertility is NOT a sin and it is NOT God's way of punishing someone. Infertility is a medical condition caused by a number of different things.

What's more, infertility doesn't mean you cannot be a parent. Adoption is always as possibility. The process isn't always easy and (take it from someone who knows) it is considerably more labor-intensive than having a biological child. And don't let anyone ever tell you that adoptive parents aren't parents in every sense of the word, because they are.

Choosing to be childless is not a sin, either. Christian couples choose to remain childless in order to be able to pursue their ministries without the distractions of family. Frank and Ella are an example of this mindset.

Frank and Ella spent thirty years as dedicated youth directors. Neither felt comfortable or working with small children or babies. Tweens and teens, however, were a different story. They poured themselves into ministering to young people this age and their efforts were highly effective.

So rather than having biological children of their own, this couple chose to 'have' dozens of children over the years; loving, teaching, and mentoring them to know and love the LORD. Other couples may choose not to have children for any number of reasons that are personal in nature; reasons that are between them and the LORD. For anyone to pass judgement on these people would be very wrong.

According to scripture God prefers we have children. Children are proof of the love between a man and a woman. Children are the hope of the future—both the future of this world and of the Church. So be fruitful and multiply; raising your children to know the LORD and that they are fearfully and wonderfully made by Him and for Him.

Chapter 4: We're Having a Baby

You've been anxiously waiting for the days and weeks to pass so that you could take a pregnancy test. The day came, you took the test, and you are on 'cloud nine' because the test came back positive. YOU ARE GOING TO HAVE A BABY!

In the days immediately following, you and your spouse shared the good news with family and close friends. You've pinched yourself (literally or figuratively speaking) a few times to remind yourself you aren't dreaming—that this is actually happening. You and your spouse have already started tossing a few names around and you have already had your first mini-panic-attack over whether or not you can go through the labor process and then actually be responsible for a helpless baby. If so, relax. All of these thoughts (and a whole lot more we're getting ready to talk about) are completely normal.

They are just part of the whole pregnancy experience. Your thoughts and worries are no different than those of any other parent-to-be, so we're going to spend the next few minutes talking about the most common thoughts and concerns of parents during those first few days and weeks following the moment you find out that you are going to have a baby.

Telling your spouse

It wasn't all that long ago women didn't have the capability to find out whether or not they were pregnant until they were at least eight weeks into the pregnancy or without going to the doctor to have blood drawn to test to see if the level of the hormone, hCG is high; indicating there is a pregnancy.

It also wasn't all that long ago expectant fathers weren't nearly as involved in the pregnancy experience or the birth of their baby as most expectant fathers are today.

Expectant fathers were usually unaware pregnancy was even a possibility until their wife shares the good news.

Today things are a lot quicker, easier, and a lot more of a joint effort. The prospective parents communicate a lot more directly about the possibility of whether or not pregnancy is possible. If, however, you are an expectant mom who wants to surprise your husband with the wonderful news, there are a number of fun ways to do so.

Give your husband a baby onesie with the logo of his favorite sports team, and a note that says 'from' your baby saying can't wait to meet you Dad, a giant cookie with your approximate due-date written in icing, or a devotional book for dads - nice.

Telling your family and close friends

Your parents, grandparents, and siblings should hear the news before the general public does.

A phone call or face-to-face visit to share your good news may be a bit 'plain', but it gets the job done. If you want to spice it up a bit try gifting grandparents with a t-shirt or mug with a grandparent saying on it is always fun. Phone calls, emails, or posts on your social media are effective and sufficient for telling friends and extended family members about your pregnancy.

Telling your employer

A close friend of mine had to go to her new boss the second day she was on the job and tell him she was pregnant. The pregnancy was something she and her husband had all but given up on happening, so learning she was going to be a mother again was an answered prayer. But it was also nerve racking. She didn't know her new employer so she had no idea how he would take the news. Thankfully he was gracious and understanding and did not treat her any differently than he did any other employee.

Telling your employer should be a priority. They need to know so that you can discuss how things like prenatal appointments and maternity leave are handled. You also need to talk to the HR person to find out what your insurance does and does not cover—what your options are regarding participating providers.

While there are some jobs that might require you to go to a limited duty status or make some special arrangements for bouts of morning sickness, being on your feet too long, or other such things. You need to remember that being pregnant is not a disease or a disability. Don't treat it as such by taking advantage of your coworkers or employer.

Choosing an OBGYN

More than likely you already have a doctor who will care for you throughout your pregnancy and who will deliver your baby. You have probably been seeing them for your yearly exams.

But there are instances in which this is not the case. If for example you have to move for a job just prior to giving birth – you will need to find a new doctor.

The whole doctor situation can be a bit unnerving. You want someone you can trust, right? Someone you feel comfortable with. Because this isn't always possible it is just one more reason for you to put your faith in the Great Physician—Jesus. He is always on-call. He will never be too busy to care for you. He knows your every need and those of your baby. He is the one you can always put your trust in and know He's got your back.

Early good prenatal care is essential

No matter who your doctor is or how and when you tell everyone else about the baby growing inside of you, the most important thing you can do for yourself and your baby is to take great care of yourself physically and emotionally.

Thankfully, most expectant moms don't have any trouble tweaking their normal lifestyle or routines once they find out they are expecting. You know—things like giving up caffeine, bouncing over rough and rocky trails on an ATV, or even putting their hobby of refinishing antique furniture on hold.

I'm here to suggest, however, that you start these things before you know you are pregnant. If you are trying to get pregnant you want to create the most welcoming, healthy, and conducive environment for your growing baby as possible.

So if you are reading this book in anticipation of the day you find out you are pregnant, start making those changes today. If you are newly-pregnant there is no question that the things I mentioned above (along with several others) are no-no's for pregnant women wanting a healthy pregnancy and healthy baby.

But if there are somethings you are in question about, don't hesitate to ask your doctor.

Congratulations! This is a wonderful, special, and amazing time in your life. Enjoy it. Make it among the happiest months of your life.

Chapter 5: The First Trimester

This book combines the biological and physiological aspects of pregnancy with the spiritual aspects of pregnancy. So in addition to learning or being reminded of what is taking place inside you (or your wife) I am also going to provide you with Scriptures of encouragement and reminders that your baby is a treasure in God's storehouse of treasures, and in spite of all that He created, He sees each and every single one of us as priceless... irreplaceable...one-of-a-kind.

Fertilization

"Do you know the time when the wild mountain goats bear young? Or can you mark when the deer gives birth? Can you number the months that they fulfill? Or do you know the time when they bear young? ~Job 39:1-2

In spite of the fact that you may be planning to try to become pregnant by charting your ovulation times, the fact remains that there is only One who knows the moment fertilization takes place and a new life begins. That One is God.

Within those first few hours when the egg and sperm join together, a new life is formed that contains chromosomes from each parent. These chromosomes determine the sex of the baby along with a host of other things – but those things I'm sure you may already know about so let's move on . . .

The earliest stages of formation

For You formed my inward parts; You covered me in my mother's womb.
~Psalm 139:13

Looking at a picture of a three week-old baby may not provide a very clear picture of what is going on inside, but wonderful things are happening.

By the end of the third week after conception, your baby's body is basically three layers of cells that are working hard to form various intricate parts of the body. The first layer of cells forms the skin, the body's nervous system, and their eyes and ears. The second layer is what grows to become the baby's heart (along with the rest of the circulatory system), their bones, muscles, and ligaments, their kidneys, and their reproductive system. The inner-most layer of cells forms the respiratory and digestive organs and systems.

A brain, spine, arms, and legs

I will praise You, for I am fearfully and wonderfully made, Marvelous are Your works, And that my soul knows very well. ~Psalm 139:14

Four weeks after your baby has been conceived, which is usually around the time most women find out they are pregnant, they are starting to develop a brain, the spinal column is forming, and arms and legs look like little buds ready to sprout to be fully infant-sized.

Your baby is growing and developing their most important parts for living a healthy, well-rounded life. This is just another reason you need to make sure you are taking proper care of yourself so that your baby receives the best of care, too.

Accepting the Child God Gives You

For the body is not one member, but many. If the foot shall say, because I am not the hand, I am not of the body; is it therefore not of the body? And if the ear shall say, Because I am not the eye, I am not of the body; is it therefore not of the body? If the whole body were an eye, where were the hearing? If the whole were hearing, where were the smelling? But now hath God set the members every one of them in the body, as it hath pleased him. ~1 Corinthians 12:14-18

Weeks five and six following conception are busy ones, to say the least. The shape of the head becomes more distinctive, as do the eyes, ears, and nose. While your baby cannot yet see, the retinas are forming; meaning and it won't be long before they can.

Fingers begin to form on the little short arms that are still yet to grow to their full length. The upper lip is formed, and the neck becomes straighter and more distinguishable.

Most amazingly of all (in my opinion, anyway) is the fact that all of this is happening to a little person about the size of a penny!

During the final weeks of the first trimester your baby's size goes from that of a penny to about the size of a credit card. By the time the first trimester comes to an end your baby also has toes, elbows, definite eyelids, buds inside the mouth that will eventually become baby teeth, red blood cells are being produced by the liver (yes, that's there, too), and their genitalia begins to make its presence known on the outside of the body.

No wonder you don't feel like your normal self

Now if God so clothes the grass of the field, which today is, and tomorrow is thrown into the oven, will He not much more clothe you, O you of little faith? "Therefore do not worry, saying, 'What shall we eat?' or 'What shall we drink?' or 'What shall we wear?' For after all these things the Gentiles seek. For your heavenly Father knows that you need all these things..
~Matthew 6:30-32

Now that you've been given a very brief and basic rundown of what is going on inside a woman's body during those first weeks of pregnancy, do you even have to ask why they don't feel like themselves? Is it any wonder that extreme fatigue is completely normal for expectant mothers, as is nausea, aka morning sickness?

These first weeks and months can be physically and emotionally exhausting. There's no doubt about that. But as a Christian you have the promise that God can and will sustain you through this time so that you can enjoy the blessings of being a steward of one of His treasures.

Chapter 6: The Second Trimester

As you enter into the second trimester of your pregnancy, you usually begin to feel better (no more morning sickness) and your energy level begins to rise. For many women, the second trimester of pregnancy is a time when they feel better than they've ever felt. They are excited about the baby's upcoming arrival. They are enjoying the fact that they are growing a baby-bump; bringing with it all sorts of positive attention and well-wishes. Thinking about names, nursery décor, and all the other fun things that go with becoming parents seem to start taking root during the second trimester.

While everything going on, on the outside is great, what's happening on the inside is even more thrilling. Let's take a look...

Diapers not needed...yet

As you do not know what is the way of the wind, Or how the bones grow in the womb of her who is with child, So you do not know the works of God who makes everything.. ~Ecclesiastes 11:5

Beginning around the eleventh week after conception (which is technically the thirteenth week of pregnancy because the two weeks between ovulation and what would have been your next period are counted) your baby begins to pee. Their pee becomes part of the amniotic fluid your baby will live in until they makes their grand appearance into the world.

Along with that major developmental milestone, your baby's bones are hardening, more red blood cells are forming in other organs, and their sex organs are becoming more distinctive.

Something new almost every day

Before I formed thee in the belly I knew thee; and before thou camest forth out of the womb I sanctified thee, and I ordained thee a prophet unto the nations. ~Jeremiah 1:5

As you progress further into your second trimester your baby starts developing more and more of the functions and characteristics they will need to live outside the womb. They develop the ability to hear, blink their eyes, and their heart is pumping around one hundred pints of blood each day. Your baby is also rolling and flipping around quite a bit, but is still too small for you to feel these movements. Don't worry, it won't be long before you do. Additionally, their digestive system is now working and they are almost as long as a dollar bill.

Reaching the halfway mark

But the very hairs of your head are all numbered. ~Matthew 10:30

During the second trimester you will hit the half-way mark of your pregnancy. It is about this time that an ultrasound can reveal to you the sex of your child (if you want to know).

Being able to recognize your baby as either a boy or a girl isn't the only significant milestone in your baby's development during this time though. Throughout the remaining weeks of the second trimester of your pregnancy you will begin to feel your baby's movements. This is one of the most exciting aspects of pregnancy. To be able to feel your baby moving around inside your body is...is...well, there really are no adequate words to fully capture the specialness of how this feels (physically or emotionally).

It is also possible for the baby's father, grandparents, or whoever else you invite, to feel the baby's movements by placing your hand on your tummy during the baby's more active times. This, too, is a very special event and a precious bonding experience for husbands and wives and for soon-to-be-dads and their unborn child.

Discovering the sex of your baby and being able to feel their movements isn't the only things that happen during these final weeks of the second trimester. There are also many significant things going on inside your baby's body.

The sound of your voice

My son, hear the instruction of thy father, and forsake not the law of thy mother: For they shall be an ornament of grace unto thy head, and chains about thy neck .~Proverbs 1:8-9

Your baby has definite times of being asleep and awake. They can even be awakened by your movements and noises outside the womb. I find this incredible, don't you!

Your baby's body is covered in the cheesy coating and a fine layer of fuzz or hair. These things both serve to keep your baby's skin from being chapped by the amniotic fluid.

Your baby's fingerprints and footprints are engraved onto their little bodies. Each one, we know, different from anyone else's every born.

Your baby can suck their thumb and recognize Mom's voice. Yes, that's right—*they know your voice before they ever see your face!*

By the end of the second trimester your baby's lungs are developing at a rapid pace; preparing them to make their grand entrance in a few months. But because the baby's lungs and their ability to suck properly are not yet fully established, it is important that you take care to keep your baby from making their entrance too soon to avoid complications. If that happens, however, just remember God is the One in Control and He has a plan for everyone including your baby.

By the time you come to the end of your second trimester your baby weighs approximately two pounds and is approximately nine inches long – and that to me is just Awesome to think about.

Chapter 7: The Third Trimester

You're almost there—'there' being the end of your pregnancy. At this point you are feeling both excited and nervous. You are getting tired of wearing maternity clothes, yet are 'certain' you'll never be able to wear anything a 'normal' woman wears again. You have days you feel energized and ready to take on the world, but then others you feel like a beached whale that can barely get one foot in front of the other. It's that whole rollercoaster effect kicking into high gear again.

This is also the point in your pregnancy when you begin getting serious about preparing the nursery, enjoy putting all those tiny little clothes in the closet and dresser drawers, and preparing for maternity leave from your job.

At this point you also need to be finalizing arrangements for childcare once you return to work—if you plan to do so. I cannot stress how important this is, because the weeks you are home with your baby after he or she arrives fly by all too quickly. In other words, you aren't going to have the time or desire to deal with this issue while on maternity leave, so it is essential you do so now.

I also want to tell you how important it is to *enjoy* these last few weeks of your pregnancy. These are special weeks in your life—weeks that cannot be replicated no matter how many children you have. Each pregnancy story is different and needs to be experienced as the miracle it truly is.

Getting ready, but not quite set to go

For we are his workmanship, created in Christ Jesus unto good works, which God hath before ordained that we should walk in them.
~Ephesians 2:10

The third and final trimester of your pregnancy is your baby's time to develop and grow into all those finishing touches that make us capable of living outside the womb. During these last few weeks your baby's hair comes in on their heads or not(it just depends on your family).

Your baby is also stretching and kicking—sometimes causing you a good deal of discomfort. For example, one mom delivered her second daughter with an extremely bruised tailbone—bruised from the inside due to the baby's near-constant kicking and jabbing –ouch! And then there are those more comical incidents surrounding the baby's movement during the last trimester. More than one expectant mom I know has had a bowl of popcorn or other snack resting on her belly, only to have it knocked off by the baby's movements.

Your baby can and will likely have hiccups; something you can feel them doing, but cannot help them with.

At the onset of the third trimester your baby will also start working quite diligently to put on weight. The added weight and layers of fat they form fill out their skin making it less wrinkled and protects their hardening bones. This protection is necessary, because even though their bones are hardening, they are still quite soft in comparison to what they will be later on. Remember—they have to be pliable enough to make it through the birth canal.

The Father's finishing touches

The spirit of God hath made me, and the breath of the Almighty hath given me life. ~Job 33:4

Thirty weeks after conception (week thirty-two of your 'official' pregnancy) your baby starts breathing practice. They are gearing up for the outside world. To this point they have breathed in and out, but it has been more instinctive than purposeful.

At this point in time the bulk of the fuzz that has covered your baby's body also begins to fall off. The degree to which this happens varies greatly in each child. As you may already know, some babies are more hairy than others when they are born. Premature babies are especially so, if born before this stage of development. The amount of baby fuzz isn't an indicator of anything being wrong with the baby. It is simply just one aspect of their unique nature showing through.

In the final weeks of gestation your baby develops the ability to detect light. They gain about an ounce of weight per day, the added weight and fat content causes their little bodies to fill out even more, and they begin positioning themselves into the birth canal.

Your doctor will likely be checking you weekly at this point to make sure everything is going as it should.

Some doctors even do an ultrasound toward the end of the pregnancy to check to make sure the umbilical cord isn't wrapped around the baby's neck, to make sure the baby's head is not so large that they feel it would be unsafe for the mother to have a vaginal delivery, and a number of other things.

It is also at this point that mothers who are having a c-section will schedule their baby's delivery. Most c-sections are scheduled to take place the week of the due date or possibly a few days prior to the due date the mother was given. This is done in an effort to avoid the baby trying to come on its own, which in most cases of mothers having C-sections, would not be a good thing.

Most C-sections are done for the sake of either the mother or child's physical condition. However, if at all possible I strongly recommend having a vaginal birth as there are many added health benefits for the baby.

Remember, the last stages of your baby's development are important to you and to them. So continue to take care of yourself and to give your baby every possible opportunity to grow and develop the way God intended them too.

Your third trimester (and pregnancy) is almost over. D-day is fast approaching.

Chapter 8: Let's Do This

At this point in your pregnancy you probably have the crib set up, you've been to childbirth classes (if you chose to take them), you have your bag packed for the hospital, and a solid birthing plan in place. You know exactly how you want things to go and you have every intention of making the birth of your child an absolutely, positively, perfectly wonderful experience.

The only thing you aren't counting on is the fact that more often than not, the best laid birthing plans fly right out the window about the time the contractions start coming around five minutes apart.

This really hurts

To the woman He said: "I will greatly multiply your sorrow and your conception; In pain you shall bring forth children; Your desire shall be for your husband, And he shall rule over you."
~Genesis 3:16

With the first baby you 'know' it's going to hurt. You've talked to other moms. You've read a few books and watched a few movies. But geez, how hard can it really be? If it was *that* bad there wouldn't be as many babies as there are. If it was *that* bad, not even sex would make it worth the 'risk'.

The thing to remember is that every women is different and every birth is different. When my wife started getting contractions I thought it was false labor and went back to sleep because I had exams the following day. However, shortly thereafter she came back in, woke me up, and said "Its Time to Go". We contacted the OBGYN and got everything we needed and headed out.

When she got to the hospital she was close to 5cm dilated. My wife no doubt is a solider and not every women could handle that as if it was no big deal but there are some.

Keep in mind my wife is just over 5' tall and weighs a little over 100lbs (not including the pregnancy weight). So if she can do it you probably can too. Just don't have any preconceived ideas about how much pain it will be because you truly don't know.

The experience of giving birth is not something you can plan for right down to your baby's first cry. There are too many variables you have no control over. Things like: where you are when your labor starts, how long the labor and delivery will take, how cooperative your baby is, how well you work with your body's natural instincts to get the job done, and the overall type of labor experience you have.

If you are reading this and think that because you are about to give birth to baby number two, don't get too smug. Every birth is different. Don't believe me? Ask any mom who has more than one child.

That thing they say about the pain being worth it...they're right

A woman, when she is in labor, has sorrow because her hour has come; but as soon as she has given birth to the child, she no longer remembers the anguish, for joy that a human being has been born into the world. ~John 16:21

I'm not going to spend a lot of time talking about the actual labor and delivery process or about the things that take place within the first few hours and days following your child's birth. Your doctor will cover all of that, and that's as it should be.

What I do want to say is that becoming a parent truly is a cause for joy and celebration. It really is the most amazing and most important thing you will ever do in this world—second only to giving your life to Christ.

So will you really forget the pain? Will the memory really go away?

The Word of God is true in all ways—including this. Though you will remember that it hurts and your memories of the event will always be there, the memories will be such that you will see the marvelous good that came from it—not the anguish and suffering you felt.

Chapter 9: Family

Welcoming a new baby into your family is news parents don't hesitate to share while having a big smile plastered across their face and heart. Think about it...how many birth announcements have you gotten that say something like, "We're as happy as we can be to announce we are now a family of three!" or "Our family is growing day by day now that baby number three has come to stay."?

Parents, grandparents, aunts, uncles, cousins should all be a part of your child's life for so many reasons. There are far too many to cover them all adequately, lets take a few minutes to cover the most important ones now...

Family provides a sense of belonging

God set up the institution of family because He knows we thrive best when we have the communion of relationships. He knows we need to be needed and need to be wanted. He knows family units and provides the sense of belonging He created us to want and need.

Family brings a sense of responsibility

Having a child changes you—or at least it should. Having a child causes you to be less selfish and more selfless. You suddenly find yourself completely and utterly responsible for another human life. You realize that what you do and how you do it affects someone else. You realize that where you go, how you act, what you say, and everything else about your life isn't just about you—it's about you and your baby.

Family becomes more important

How many new parents have you heard say something to the effect that when their baby was born their own parents (the baby's grandparents) suddenly became wiser and smarter than they'd ever been before?

News flash! The grandparents didn't suddenly become anything (other than grandparents). The wisdom and knowledge was there before the baby was born. But when faced with the awesome and daunting task of actually being a parent themselves, well….

The role of grandparent, aunt or uncle can be a precious resource in the lives of children and their parents. For a child, these extended family members can be sounding boards, people who have time when parents don't, an added source of encouragement and unconditional love, someone to teach them skills their parents don't have, someone to just hang out with, someone to whom they can give back all of these things, and someone they can look up to as an example of faith.

Those of you who have families that can bring these things into your child's life should be thankful for the blessing of family. It is something you should not take for granted and should not deprive your child of.

Those of you who do not have family to lean on and glean from, do not have to miss out completely. You can 'adopt' a family in your church. There are undoubtedly people as hungry for a family as you are.

Family isn't always about blood and DNA. It's about exhibiting the kind of love that says "I love you just because". Never forget those that claim the name of Jesus Christ and claim His Blood are Adopted into the Family of God – So You are NEVER Alone!.

Chapter 10: Children are the Future

Babies and children just add that something extra into a family's dynamics. They bring a sense of innocence, wonder, fun, and youthfulness into a home. Children also give us purpose—or at least they should. Being a parent should make you stand a little taller on the 'ladder' of integrity. They should make you think on your words before you speak them; making sure they are honest, kind, and fair. Children should make you walk a straighter path; working hard, spending your money wisely, being honest and forthright, and setting a solid example of how to live. Children should make you desire to know God more fully and to teach them to know God on a personal level, too, because children are the future of society and of the Church.

One of the most heart-rending statements I've ever heard went something like this: The worst possible feeling a parent could have is the feeling that they might not spend eternity with their children in heaven.

Ouch! That cuts deep, doesn't it? As parents we need to be mindful of the fact that we are responsible for raising our children to know the LORD and to have a desire to seek his purpose for their lives.

That being said, you need to remember that your purpose is to raise them to know these things—not live their lives for them.

We have this Promise from God . . . .

Train up a child in the way he should go, And when he is old he will not depart from it.
~Proverbs 22:6

While none of us are perfect; meaning we all make parenting mistakes (and plenty of them), if we do our job to raise our children as directed by God in the Bible, we have nothing to worry about. You can do it as God fearing Parents that seek the Living God and honor Him by following the Word of God on how to raise your children.

Don't let things discourage or frighten you, along the way. There will always be ups and downs in life but in all things God is an ever present help in a time of need – Trust in Him, Allow His Word to inspire you to become a great parent who raises awesome kids.

Do as we are told in Lamentations 2:19...

Arise, cry out in the night: in the beginning of the watches pour out thine heart like water before the face of the Lord: lift up thy hands toward him for the life of thy young children that faint for hunger in the top of every street.

In reading this book you have either learned or have been reminded of the fact that being a parent isn't just something physical that you do. Being a parent is also a spiritual act—one that God intends to be a spiritual act of worship aimed at Him.

God knows that when we see our children as the priceless treasures they are we will love, nurture, and cherish them in such a way that glorifies God.

Parenting Special Needs Children

A Christian Guide to Parenting Children
with ADHD, Autism, Asperger's, and
other Psychological, Behavioral, or
Physiological Disorders

By: Patrick Baldwin

Prelude

Having worked for close to 20 years with those in our society that are considered some of the most vulnerable, I wanted to write this book to offer Biblical Guidance for the Christian Parent.

Often times we may become overwhelmed with the thoughts, responsibilities, and day to day grind that having a special needs child can bring to your life. It is critical to see Your Child through the Eyes of God and to Keep Your Focus on Jesus Christ along the Way.

I truly Pray that this book will be a Blessing to You and Your Family and hope that You will share it with other Christian Parents who may be also dealing with the challenges of Parenting a Special Needs Child.

God Bless You

Chapter 1: You Are Going to be the Parent of a Special Needs Child

When we see the little line on the pregnancy test saying there is a baby growing inside of you, the last thing you probably think about (or one of the last things) is whether or not your baby will have special needs when it comes to their physical, mental, or emotional wellbeing.

You aren't thinking about whether or not you will be able to afford special equipment they might need to live. You aren't thinking about what your insurance will and won't cover and what kind of help you can get to make up the difference. You aren't thinking about whether or not your house will 'work' for a wheelchair, if your boss will allow you to work from home or how you will juggle work and five or six doctor's appointments a month (or possibly in a week).

You aren't thinking about the fact that your baby—the one you've just 'met'—is one of the millions of children in this country that will receive some form of special education when he or she goes to school. And that's providing he or she can go to school.

No, you aren't thinking about those things at all. You are thinking about whether the baby is a boy or girl, when the due date will be, who to share the happy news with first (other than your spouse, of course), and you even start rolling possible names around in your mind. In other words, your thoughts are focused on the joy that comes from bringing a new baby into this world.

Well guess what? Bringing a new baby into this world regardless of whether or not they have special needs *is* a joy. Each and every tiny little life that takes their first breath after working their way into this world is a cause for celebration and joy *because* we are all fearfully and wonderfully made by the LORD God, our Creator.

Nevertheless, learning your child has special needs—whether you find out prior to or immediately after their birth, or a few months or years down the road—is difficult. Your love for your child instinctively wants them to be 'normal'. You don't want them to have to struggle. You don't want them to have to go through the experience of feeling different from the rest of the kids or to experience the loneliness often felt from being left out of so many things kids like to do. You don't want to see the hurt in their eyes and know their hearts are breaking when they are made fun of or ostracized by their peers.

What's more, you can't help worrying about how their condition or circumstances is going to affect your life and the lives of other family members. And then you start feeling guilty for feeling and thinking that way; making you even more anxious.

Am I right? You know I am. But the GREAT news is that it is perfectly normal and okay to feel and think these things—as long as you are near enough to Jesus to dump it all at His feet so that he can replace all of those things with what you need in order to do the very special job you have been given by God to do.

That's right—being given the responsibility of parenting a child with special needs is NOT a form of discipline or punishment. Instead, God is saying, "I have a special job for you because your heart's capacity to love and nurture is above and beyond what is normal. I created you with the ability to see beyond the obvious into the heart and soul of one of my children, so I need you to raise them up for me."

We see this truth in the Gospel of John, chapter nine, when Jesus heals a man who had been born blind. Jesus and His disciples were coming into a village when they saw the man, who was most likely begging in front of the marketplace or along the road that led into the village.

When the disciples saw that he was blind, they asked Jesus whether it was he or his parents whose sin had caused him to be born blind. (That's the punishment 'thing' I just mentioned.)

Jesus immediately replied that neither the sins of the man nor those of his parents had caused his blindness. And then in the next breath, Jesus added these words: Jesus answered, "Neither this man nor his parents sinned, but that the works of God should be revealed in him..." (John 9:3 NKJV)

Did you get that? The man's blindness wasn't a curse or punishment. He had been born blind so that he could be an instrument through which Jesus' holiness and power could be displayed. He was literally a partner in Jesus' ministry!

So while parenting a special-needs child maybe wasn't what you anticipated doing as a parent, and while you may feel completely overwhelmed and even terrified at the prospect of doing so, don't let these feelings rob your child of the joy he or she deserves to feel in your touch and see in your eyes that says, "I'm so glad you are mine." And whatever you do, don't let these feelings rob you of the joy you deserve to experience in becoming and being a parent and of the blessing of being God's partner in showing the world just how Holy and Mighty He is.

Bible Verses to Encourage You

And not only that, but we also glory in tribulations, knowing that tribulation produces perseverance; 4 and perseverance, character; and character, hope. ~Romans 5:3-4

And the Lord said unto him, who hath made man's mouth? or who maketh the dumb, or deaf, or the seeing, or the blind? have not I the Lord? ~Exodus 4:11

For thou hast possessed my reins: thou hast covered me in my mother's womb. I will praise thee; for I am fearfully and wonderfully made: marvelous are thy works; and that my soul knoweth right well. ~Psalm 139:13-14

Lo, children are an heritage of the Lord: and the fruit of the womb is his reward. ~Psalm 127:3

Chapter 2: Guarding Your Heart, Soul, Mind, and Strength

You can have all the joy, joy, joy, joy down in your heart, in your head, and bubbling up out of your soul imaginable but that won't erase the fact that parenting a special-needs child is hard work. It is physically exhausting, mentally and emotionally draining, time-consuming, and often times very, very lonely. I think it's safe to say that this is one of those things about which your grandma would say, "The most worthwhile jobs we do are the hardest jobs we do".

Because there is so much required of you, it is important that you take care of yourself. *Good* care of yourself. This is something many parents of special-needs children don't do a very well. Generally speaking, parents put the needs of their children in front of their own needs—as we should in many instances, but not *all.*

And when you take into consideration that the demands on your life because of the increased needs of your child…. I guess you could say that parents of special-needs children have some special needs of their own.

What you are about to read is a list of things you need to be doing for YOURSELF. Don't make excuses and the words "I can't" are not allowed—not even in your head or under your breath. Taking good care of yourself is key to doing your job to the best of your ability and key to knowing you, too, are fearfully and wonderfully made (Psalm 139).

1: Spend time in the Word daily

Ten or fifteen minutes spent reading the Bible each day is food for the soul, body, and mind. Don't just focus on the Psalms or the Gospels—books of the Bible that are usually viewed as the 'feel good' books of the Bible. While you *do* need to make them part of your Bible study, they shouldn't be the only part.

When you spend time in the books of history you become more grounded and sure of the fact that God does have a plan.

The books of Job and Ecclesiastes humble you and remind you that the most important things in life aren't things and that God really does have the whole world (including you and your child) in His hands.

The book of Esther gives us an extra dose of courage and reminds us that our ultimate purpose is to bring Glory to God through all we do and say.

The prophets don't spare words. They tell it like it is when it comes to reminding us that we are all sinners. But they are equally eloquent when it comes to reminding us of God's abundant love and mercy—love and mercy we can draw on every…single…day.

James and most of Paul's letters are the books that keep us on the straight and narrow. They define Christian character, warn us of the consequences for living outside of God's laws and expectations, and reaffirm the promises of heaven in all its glory when we abide in Jesus Christ.

Read God's Word. Apply it to your life. Let it speak to you. Let it change you.

2: Pray

One of the biggest concerns and complaints of parents with special-needs children is that they don't have many people they can talk to who really 'gets' it. Not on a regular basis, that is, because the parents who *do* 'get' it are as busy as they are. But God always hears and He is always available. No, He's not someone you can sit around the table with over a cup of coffee or someone you can chat with while you take a lap or two around the block.

But He *is* there, He *does* listen, and He *does* care.

You also need to know (or be reminded of the fact) that your conversations are not one-sided. God responds to you. He responds by:

- Telling the Holy Spirit what to say to you (Jon 16:13)
- Speaking to you through the Scriptures
- Providing answers through your conversations and interactions with others – Something called Confirmation.

In 1 Thessalonians 5:17 we are told to pray without ceasing. If you do that, you'll also be conversing with God nonstop.

3: Eat a healthy diet

God created our bodies to operate at optimum efficiency and capacity when we feed our bodies a steady diet of the food He created for us to eat. Meat, fruits, veggies, dairy products, grains…the things He created to fuel our bodies.

Sure there are exceptions—food allergies and personal tastes, for example. But for the most part you really need to make sure your diet consists primarily of foods free of chemicals, dyes, and processing.

If you are still looking for things like chips, blooming onions, mocha latte caramel coffee with an extra shot of caffeine, diet soda, and seven-layer lasagna on the list of best foods, you can stop. They aren't there. They never will be.

Eating a healthy diet keeps your body working the way it should. Your heart is healthier. Your body doesn't produce a lot of bad fat for you to carry around. You think more clearly. You reduce your risk of getting things like heart disease, diabetes, kidney failure, and bone and joint disorders due to carrying around too much weight. You have more energy. Your immune system does a better job of fighting off colds and the flu.

Question: What's not to like about the benefits of eating a healthy diet?

Answer: Nothing. So do it!

4: Get plenty of exercise

If your child has physical limitations that require you to bathe them, dress them, and help them move from one place to another, you are undoubtedly getting quite a bit of physical activity.

But that doesn't mean you don't need to get twenty minutes or so of walking, yoga, aerobics, or whatever else you like to do at least three days a week.

If at all possible, you should also set aside an hour or two each week for more rigorous exercise. A few possible options include: Water aerobics, tennis, volleyball, working out at the gym, swimming laps, or anything else you enjoy that gets your heart pumping.

The physical benefits of exercise go without saying and should be reason enough to make sure you get this time each week. But the physical benefits are just the tip of the proverbial iceberg. So what are the benefits?

- Exercise increases oxygen to the brain; helping you clear your head and think more rationally and clearly.

- Exercise releases endorphins. Endorphins are hormones that send messages to the brain that tell the brain to think positive thoughts. Endorphins also lessen our perception of pain. They intercept the signals from our nerves and send the message to the brain that it doesn't hurt as bad as 'all that'.
- Exercise keeps your weight in check and your heart healthy.
- Exercise gives you some much-deserved time off from your responsibilities as a parent. Even if it is only for a few minutes a day, it is worth it.
- Exercise boosts your immune system. This is actually one of the top two or three reasons parents of special-needs children take time to exercise.

- After all, when parents get sick (especially Mom) chaos at home can quickly ensue. So remember... "An ounce of prevention is worth a pound of cure".
- Some forms of exercise provide you with a social outlet. Even if you and a friend take several laps around the block or park, it still counts as time you can enjoy conversations without interruptions.

5: Date nights and marriage protection

Couples with children—no matter how many and no matter what their needs are—all run the risk of letting parenting, work, money-matters, and everything else push their marriage and its wellbeing to the backburner. But when you add the stresses of raising a special-needs child to the mix, the chances of this happening increase significantly.

The financial burdens that come from having a special-needs child are often very heavy to bear. The primary caregiver (usually Mom) doesn't have a lot of time to just sit and talk. She doesn't always have the luxury of prioritizing how her time is spent. That is usually done for her out of sheer necessity. That's why as parents of a special-needs child you need to make conscious and consistent effort to have couple time free of ANY talk about home, money, the kids, or anything else that pertains to your daily routine. You need to make a conscious effort to make romantic gestures and let your spouse know they are second only to God.

What? But...our child needs me to do…. Who has time for romance? And since my life pretty much revolves around making sure our kids are taken care of, there's not really much else to talk about.

Oh, but there is. There is plenty to talk about:

- Make plans for a weekend getaway…just the two of you
- Talk about an upcoming event at church
- Talk about some things you would like to make time to do for yourself
- Make plans for a family weekend
- Talk about current events
- Recall memories from your dating years and the early years of your marriage
- Talk about the reasons you love one another
- Talk about long-range goals for your marriage and family
- Talk about something funny you saw on television or at the grocery store
- Make a list of ideas of things you can do to keep your marriage fresh and thriving…and then start doing the things on that list

There are several other things you need to make sure you don't neglect to do in order to keep your marriage safe and fresh. These things include:

- Worshipping together.
- Serving together in your church and community.
- Letting your children see and hear you being (appropriately) affectionate with each other.
- Not allowing your children to play you against one another.
- Making sure you kiss each other good morning, hello, goodbye, and goodnight.
- Telling each other "I love you" every single day.
- Not neglecting your appearance—your 'Sunday best' isn't always necessary, but baggy pants, t-shirts, and a messy-hair-don't-care look doesn't say much about the way you feel about yourself.

- And if you don't care about yourself, it's hard for other people to do so.
- Taking care of your body.
- Showing an interest in your spouse's job (in and away from the home).
- Making their friends feel welcome in your home.
- Respecting their need for 'me' time and giving them that luxury.
- Making sure 'me' time and 'friend' time never add up to more than the time you spend with your spouse and your family.
- Living with the attitude of submission (for wives) and sacrificial love and leadership (for husbands) as directed in the New Testament book of Ephesians.

7: Fellowship

You need fellowship. You need to spend time with your peers; studying God's Word, socializing, enjoying recreational activities and outings, and just hanging out. Just being yourself.

While there is nothing wrong with part of this fellowship coming in the form of support groups or play groups with other parents of special-needs children, this should not be your *only* outlet. These groups are can be very beneficial—a lifeline for many of you—but you need to be able to fellowship in ways that address *your* needs and interests…not your child's.

Don't think this is being selfish. It's not. By giving yourself this time you are giving your family a better and you—an energized, more confident, refreshed you. So don't feel guilty about taking some time for a Bible study, a weekly game of golf or tennis, meeting up for coffee and fellowship, a book club, or some other group where you can share your passion for your hobby with others who feel the same.

The amount of time you allow yourself isn't a number that is set in stone. There is no magic number that guarantees your needs will be met. For some, an afternoon, evening, or possibly an entire day (or most of it, anyway) a week is doable. For others, though, an hour or two a week is a priceless and treasured gift that happens only with a great deal of planning, preparation, and help from others.

Speaking of help...

8: Ask for help

You can't do this on your own. Physically...emotionally...mentally...you need help and support.

The help and support you receive can come from a number of different resources. Some of these resources exist solely for the purpose of helping parents of special-needs children and the children themselves. Other sources of help are people who love and care about you and want to be the hands and feet of Jesus in your life. And you need to let them do that.

Bobby and Shannon were the parents of six year-old twins and a three year-old born without hands—his arms stop just below his elbows. Bobby, Shannon, and all three children are completely comfortable with their life. Even the twins are a great help when it comes to feeding, dressing, and playing with their little brother.

But they are hesitant to leave their son in anyone's care other than his grandparents when they came to visit or the physical therapist they met with a couple of hours a week. So other than these two hours a week and four or five visits a year from grandparents, Bobby and Shannon took no time for just the two of them.

Friends from church have offered to take all three of the kids on numerous occasions, but Shannon always made an excuse. Thanks, but no thanks, was the message she conveyed. But then one day, a middle-aged woman at church asked Shannon a question that stopped her in her tracks. She asked, " Why do you insist on keeping people from doing what Jesus wants them to do?"

"Excuse me," Shannon asked back, somewhat offended. "What do you mean?"

"People in this church, including me, want to be part of your family and want you to be part of ours. We want to minister to your family, get to know you and your kids, let you know you have people who love and care about you. We want to live and love the way Jesus told us to, but you won't let us," was the woman's answer.

Shannon didn't know what to say. She'd never thought about it like that before. She was so focused on not wanting to appear to be a charity case or give people a reason to think they needed to feel sorry for them and their son, that she had completely forgotten that Jesus calls us to love and serve one another. This woman was right! By not accepting their offers for help and fellowship, they were robbing these people of opportunities to be like Jesus. And what's more, they were robbing themselves of the blessings that come with being a part of a family of believers.

From that day on Shannon and Bobby were more than happy to take people up on their offers to babysit so they could have date nights. And they were equally happy to return the favor by doing the same for other young families in the church. Josephine (the woman who talked to Shannon) and her husband became surrogate grandparents to their children, and relationships were built that will undoubtedly last a lifetime.

Today Shannon and Bobby are the parents for four and grandparents to two. They are also in charge of a parent's night out ministry at their church, because they know what it is like to need help AND they know how important it is for others to be able to offer it.

Besides your church family, other possible resources for help include:

- Healthcare agencies
- Playgroups for children with physical disabilities
- Daycare facilities that cater to children with special needs
- Friends and neighbors
- Support groups (for emotional and mental help you need)

9: Me time

In addition to the time you spend with just your spouse and time spent with your friends and peers, you need to have a few minutes of 'me' time every day. Thirty minutes or so each day to do whatever you want to do by yourself. Take a walk. Soak in the bathtub. Read a book. Bake cookies. Shoot some hoops. Watch television without interruption. Surf the web. Catch up on social media. Do your nails. Take a nap. Whatever you enjoy doing…do it.

The purpose of this time of solitude is to allow you to clear your head and not think about anyone or anything but yourself and what you are doing. This is your time to dream, plan, rest, relax, and even be a bit selfish.

Taking this time each day is so important. Knowing you have this time to look forward to each day helps you keep things in the proper perspective. It prevents you from feeling like you've lost your identity as an individual.

You are God's child. You are a spouse. You are a parent. You are an instrument of God's plan. Your body is the temple of the Holy Spirit. You cannot be and do these things if you are not practicing good self-care, so do it. It is your duty to yourself, your family, and to your God.

Bible Verses to Encourage You

It is vain for you to rise up early, to sit up late, to eat the bread of sorrows: for so he giveth his beloved sleep. ~Psalm 127:2

*I will both lie down in peace, and sleep;
For You alone, O Lord, make me dwell in safety.
~Psalm 4:8*

For I have satiated the weary soul, and I have replenished every sorrowful soul. ~Jeremiah 31:25

*There remaineth therefore a rest to the people of God. For he that is entered into his rest, he also hath ceased from his own works, as God did from His.
~Hebrews 4:9-10*

Chapter 3: True Love is Devoid of All Pride

Every parent's desire is to make their child's life good, happy, pleasant, and as carefree as possible. And why not? Isn't that just part of what loving someone is all about? But when you have a child with special needs, your quest to give these things to your child usually comes with a few (or a lot) more challenges.

Every parent is charged by God with the task of keeping their children safe and healthy, providing them with food, clothing, and shelter, and loving them unconditionally; nurturing and cherishing them for the treasure they are. Additionally, parents are responsible for raising their children to:

- Learn to be confident and comfortable with who they are
- Know that we are to be God-pleasers...not people-pleasers
- Recognize sin for what it is and rise above it

- To strive to achieve their goals and dreams

But again, children with special needs have to work a little harder to get the job done, and as their parent, *you* have to work a little harder to help them. Your success in doing so depends on your ability to set aside any prideful feelings you have—consciously or subconsciously.

Denial is not uncommon when you first learn that your child has special needs. These feelings are not necessarily evidence of shame or embarrassment. More often than not they stem from guilt, concern, and apprehension.

- Did I do something...or not do something that caused this?
- Will my child be able to enjoy at least some of the things a child should?
- Can I be the parent my child needs and deserves?

The reason for the feelings isn't necessarily important. What *is* important is that you set them aside for the sake of everyone involved. Don't let pride keep you from dong what is best for your child.

Early intervention

Denial has been the reason for many children's conditions and disabilities to go undiagnosed as soon as they could and should be. If your child isn't diagnosed as having special needs, then the problem isn't really there, right? Wrong! Early intervention often makes the difference in how severely their disability affects their life (and yours) and the degree to which they can function.

Parents, pretending or burying your head in the sand accomplishes nothing good. So don't deny your child every chance possible to be high-functioning and/or to receive therapy that allows them to be more mobile and independent. Get help at the first sign that a problem exists.

Your pediatrician will be able to connect you with available resources and information for your particular situation. Make use of them.

Living realistically

Once you know what your child's condition is and what their needs are and will be you need to listen intently and carefully to those who can point you in the right direction to get you and your child the help available to you. When meeting with therapists, doctors, and anyone else involved in your child's care, you might not always like what you hear. Sometimes parents feel the plan of action isn't aggressive enough. Some feel it is too aggressive. And some think the medical community is too pessimistic in their outlook. These are the parents that believe if their child tries hard enough they can overcome their disability.

EXAMPLE: Jared's mom was thoroughly convinced that putting her son in a classroom for special-needs students that he would never reach his full potential. She believed that if he was in a traditional classroom setting he would work harder to be on a level 'playing field' with the rest of the class.

The problem with this line of thinking is that by putting expectations on Jared he simply cannot meet makes him feel bad about himself and causes him to doubt his ability to succeed. It's like giving a five year-old keys to the car and expecting them to be able to drive.

Your child has enough to deal with because of their special needs. Don't add to that by trying to make them someone they are not and by insinuating that you are ashamed of them or that who they are is not reason enough to love them with your whole heart. Accept the fact that they have limitations. Accept what those limitations are. Put them in a position to excel to the best of their ability. Celebrate their accomplishments. Love them for who they are.

Be your child's advocate and biggest fan

Today's children are only the second or third generation of children to not be hidden away or ignored just because they have special needs. Prior to this, children with special needs were considered to be disposable and less valuable than their 'normal' peers. Children with special needs and disabilities were often placed in institutions where they did little more than exist. Others were kept at home, but were not allowed to go to school and had little or no social interaction. Think: Boo Radley in *To Kill a Mockingbird*.

Thankfully, though, not every parent 'back then' thought or felt that way…

Neal and Bonita knew something was wrong with their second-born son, Gary, before he turned six months old. He wasn't meeting the developmental milestones for babies his age.

But in those days and in their small town, it wasn't easy to get a correct diagnosis. When they did, the words they heard were MULTIPLE SCLEROSIS.

Neal and Bonita were encouraged to put Gary in a 'home' where he could live out his days (which they were told would be less than twenty years) peacefully and out of the harsh and unaccepting public eye. But they didn't want to put their son away. They knew God didn't make a mistake when he made Gary. They knew he was as treasured and loved as anyone else God created. They also knew that every child with special needs was one of God's precious treasures, too. So with nothing but a determination and passion for wanting to help Gary and others like him to reach their full potential, Neal and Bonita recruited teachers and people who practiced a trade to work in what would now be called a sheltered workshop.

Gary is now an eighty year-old man who has never walked on his own, never ran, played catch, or spoken a word that is understandable by an 'untrained' ear. But he *has* appeared before three different presidents of the United States to champion for the rights of people with disabilities, gone to Europe to compete in the Special Olympics, won multiple gold and silver medals in the same, accumulated dozens of bowling trophies, and encouraged countless people just by being himself. But these things were possible only because his parents were his biggest fans and they championed for him with relentless energy, passion, and love.

Don't let anyone make your child feel worthless and unlovable. Believe in them and do whatever you can to make sure they are given every possible and feasible opportunity to reach their full potential.

Bible Verses to Encourage You

For I know the thoughts that I think toward you, saith the Lord, thoughts of peace, and not of evil, to give you a future and a hope. ~Jeremiah 29:11

Now unto Him that is able to do exceeding abundantly above all that we ask or think, according to the power that worketh in us... ~Ephesians 3:20

For we are His workmanship, created in Christ Jesus unto good works, which God hath before ordained that we should walk in them. ~Ephesians 2:10

Chapter 4: Overcoming the Educational Obstacles

Back in the day there was an ad campaign targeting high schoolers in an effort to convince them to pursue a college education. The campaign's slogan was, "A mind is a terrible thing to waste". And it's true, a mind *is* a terrible thing to waste—and that means your child, too.

Depending on where you live, your child's school may or may not be equipped to offer your child the educational resources they need and deserve. This is not something you should waste time being angry or bitter about. In most cases the lack of resources is due to a lack of money and/or a lack of qualified teachers in the district—neither of which will be changed by your anger or bitterness. Instead, be pro-active and take matters into your own hands. Instead of wasting your time and energy, put it to use by either becoming the resources your child needs or by going beyond the walls of the school to get them.

Here are some possible ways you might do that:

Depending on your child's special needs you might consider homeschooling your child. Or better yet, consider forming a homeschool coop with other special need's parents. This has proven to be especially helpful to both parents and students with needs such as dyslexia, mild autism, sensory problems, auditory processing disorder, and a variety of delayed development issues. Educating your child in this type of environment allows them to:

- Learn in a less congested environment with fewer distractions and risks of over-stimulation and more personalized attention
- Feel safer and more accepted among their peers
- Receive instruction and training at a pace and in a format that will allow them to thrive and excel

As for parents, working together shares the workload, provides a community of support and encouragement, and it allows you to know you are giving your child the learning environment most conducive to their learning style and capabilities.

Hire a tutor. Homeschooling on any level is not always possible. And quite frankly, it is not always the best route to take. Depending on your child's needs and the resources they have available in their school, you may find that by hiring a tutor your child will be able to stay on course with the mainstream student population. You don't need to go through a professional service to find a good tutor, though. Retired teachers, teachers who have opted to stay home with their own children, but who are willing to tutor a few hours a week, or college students in need of extra money are all great resources. A tutor gives your child the one-on-one they so often need to get them over the hump and to give them the moral support and encouragement to keep trying.

Specialized schools are available in some areas—usually large cities. These are somewhat expensive, however, but *do* offer the best in special-needs education. If you live near one of these schools don't let the price tag scare you. Funding is sometimes available through scholarship programs or organizations to aid and assist children with special needs.

Public schooling is free and available to children with mild to moderately-severe special needs. Many public schools have excellent programs for children with learning disabilities and a staff of loving, caring, and dedicated teachers. Often time's public schools also offer and allow personal aides or assistants for special-needs students. The job of a personal aide/assistant is to be their student's constant companion throughout the day; assisting them in whatever ways they need assistance.

Some of the things they might do include:

- Reading to them if they cannot read but can comprehend
- Signing for the deaf
- Writing for those that cannot write but are fully able to comprehend and can speak the answers
- Feeding and other personal care

No matter what educational obstacles you encounter or what path you choose for your child, remember...a mind is a terrible thing to waste.

Bible Verses to Encourage You

How much better is it to get wisdom than gold! and to get understanding rather to be chosen than silver! ~Proverbs 16:16

Take firm hold of instruction, do not let go; Keep her, for she is your life.
~Proverbs 4:13

Give instruction to a wise man, and he will be yet wiser: teach a just man, and he will increase in learning. ~Proverbs 9:9

Chapter 5: We Are Family

When asked what challenges a special-needs child brings to the dynamics of a family, the answers are all over the map.

- "I don't think of my child's needs as something that challenges our family," one parent said. "Being a family means seeing one another as equally valuable and loving one another for who we are. So if who we are, is someone who needs help eating or who cannot play ball, then so be it."
- "I find myself working harder than I really need to sometimes to make things equal for my kids. Sometimes I feel guilty about spending more time with my daughter because of her needs, but then God reminds me that not having to do those things for my boys is a good thing."

- "It is challenging. My now-seven year-old was three when an accident left her with some physical disabilities and mild learning disabilities. I was expecting our second child at the time, so adjusting to all the changes in our routine and life in general really did keep me from enjoying my new baby. I am constantly second-guessing myself in regards to how good a mom I am to each of them."
- "I leave for work every morning knowing my wife is on a non-stop schedule. I feel guilty for being gone so much, but our son's medical expenses are over the top. We'll never be able to see the light at the end of the tunnel. We would like to have another child, but don't know how in the world we could handle two.

- We want to know what it's like to parent a child that doesn't need round the clock care (or close to it). We want to know what it's like to go to our kid's ball game or dance recital. Is that so bad or wrong?"
- We have two boys in school and our four year-old son is low-functioning autistic. The six and nine year old boys are great with him at home, but I've noticed lately they get embarrassed when Judson acts out in public and they say things like, "Can't you just take us and Mom and Judson stay home?" Or "Judson can't do that, so why does he have to come?" I know some of that is natural, but right now I'm really struggling with how to teach my boys to love their brother for who he is and to love him like they love each other."

I could say all sorts of things on how I feel or what I think on how to handle the possible challenges a special-needs child can bring to your family. But what I think and how I feel aren't important. What is important is what God has to say on the subject of family unity…regardless of the physical, mental, or emotional issues that might be present. So take a few minutes to let God's Word soak into your heart and mind. Share these verses with your spouse, your children, and even your extended family members in an effort to remind them that we are ALL created in the image of God and are ALL equally loved and valued by him.

Bible Verses to Encourage You

Love suffers long and is kind; love does not envy; love does not parade itself, is not puffed up; does not behave rudely, does not seek its own, is not provoked, thinks no evil; does not rejoice in iniquity, but rejoices in the truth; bears all things, believes all things, hopes all things, endures all things ~1 Corinthians 13:4-7 (NKJV)

We love him, because he first loved us.
~1 John 4:19

Better is a dry morsel with quietness,
Than a house full of feasting with strife.
~Proverbs 17:1

For as we have many members in one body, but all the members do not have the same function, so we, being many, are one body in Christ, and individually members of one another. ~Romans 12:4-5

For the body is not one member, but many. If the foot shall say, because I am not the hand, I am not of the body; is it therefore not of the body? And if the ear shall say, because I am not the eye, I am not of the body; is it therefore not of the body? If the whole body were an eye, where were the hearing? If the whole were hearing, where were the smelling? But now hath God set the members every one of them in the body, as it hath pleased him. ~1 Corinthians 12:15-18

Chapter 6: Let Your "Light" Shine

Remember reading about Neal and Bonita and how they refused to stifle their son, Gary's potential in time when that was the norm for kids like Gary? Thankfully things are much different today.

Today parks have playgrounds for children with even the most severe disabilities.

Today public buildings have rams and entryways that are accessible to people in a wheelchair.

Today public restrooms are equipped with facilities with enough room to maneuver around in and with sinks, toilets, etc. placed at the right height.

Today even campground shower houses have wheelchair-accessible showers.

Today parking lots provide spaces for vehicles with special-needs drivers or passengers.

Today special-needs children can grow up to be special-needs adults who contribute to society in a positive manner by working, volunteering, and just living life to the fullest.

All of these things are definitely improvements over what used to be, but that doesn't mean life for families of special-needs children is not without its share of obstacles in their communities and their social lives.

When it comes to meeting and overcoming the challenges of special-needs children and their families in the community and on the social 'scene', you need to respond the same way you should when it comes to your child's education. You need to be a pro-active advocate instead of an angry, bitter parent. And the best way to do this is to help the world see what an amazing and precious person your child is.

Proverbs 31:8 (NKJV) says: *Open your mouth for the speechless, In the cause of all who are appointed to die.* So do it! Open your mouth, use your hands to open doors, your feet to walk through them, and your mind to think of ways to help your child be a part of the world around them. Don't hide their light under a basket. Let them shine for all those around them to see...and be blessed.

- Attend church and let your child be involved in the youth program to the extent they are capable of. Be willing to act as a chaperone for youth events so that your child can participate.
- Volunteer with your child. Taking their specific needs into consideration, consider participating in walk-a-thons (or wheel-a-thons, if necessary). Fill shoe boxes with gifts for other children. Ring the Salvation Army bells. Hand out personal care bags to the homeless. Visit a nursing home together.
- Join a play group.

- Visit the park on a regular basis.
- Enroll your child in swimming lessons, bowling lessons, or some other type of activity they are capable of participating in. *Many of these activities/lessons offer special lessons for children with various handicaps.
- Join 4-H, scouts, or another similar type of organization.
- Go to the weekly story hour at your library.
- Participate in free movie nights, craft-making events, kid-friendly lectures and demonstrations, etc. offered in your community.
- Go for ice cream or an occasional dinner at a favorite family pizza place or restaurant.
- Get them involved with Special Olympics.

The "Bible Verses to Encourage You" segments in previous chapters have already listed Exodus 4:11 and Psalm 139:13-14, but I want us to look at them again because they are important reminders to everyone that God creates each of us in his image and with a distinct set of purposes in mind. Special-needs children are not mistakes. God doesn't make mistakes. Special-needs children are special-*purposes* children and as their parents you need to help them accomplish those purposes in this world.

Bible Verses to Encourage You

And the Lord said unto him, who hath made man's mouth? or who maketh the dumb, or deaf, or the seeing, or the blind? have not I the Lord? ~Exodus 4:11

For thou hast possessed my reins: thou hast covered me in my mother's womb. I will praise thee; for I am fearfully and wonderfully made: marvelous are thy works; and that my soul knoweth right well. ~Psalm 139:13-14

But indeed, O man, who are you to reply against God? Will the thing formed say to Him who formed it, "Why have you made me like this?" ~Romans 9:20

Chapter 7: Dealing With Special Social and Communication Needs

Children with social and communication special needs are those with autism, Asperger, and ADHD (as well as a few others). But then you already know that, don't you? You know that your child has difficulties interacting socially and communicating their thoughts and needs.

The severity of these conditions varies widely from person to person. In some children it is a matter of controlling their intake of certain foods and providing them with a structured environment so that they don't feel (and act) like a loose cannon. But for others, the problem is much more intense. Some children cannot speak or communicate on any level. Some children cannot handle even slight changes in their routine without becoming unsettled and sometime nearly impossible to manage or console. But again, you already know these things.

What you don't know…or need to be reminded of is that neither you nor your child is alone in the struggles you are facing to deal with life as you know it. God is ever-present.

His presence is visible in the words of the Bible:

He healeth the broken in heart, and bindeth up their wounds. ~Psalm 147:3

It is of the Lord's mercies that we are not consumed, because His compassions fail not. They are new every morning: great is thy faithfulness. The Lord is my portion, saith my soul; therefore will I hope in Him. The Lord is good unto them that wait for Him, to the soul that seeketh him. ~Lamentations 3:22-25

But God commendeth His love toward us, in that, while we were yet sinners, Christ died for us. ~Romans 5:8

Another means by which God proves His presence is in providing resources and counsel for you and your child. Because God has worked through others, we know that parents of children with autism and ADHD can help their child when they:

- Provide a consistent routine and schedule for their child
- Make home a safe, fun, and hazard-free place to be
- Make time for fun; doing things THEY enjoy doing
- Reward positive behavior
- Discover their child's triggers for tantrums and melt-downs and then take necessary actions and precautions
- Know the child's sensitivities (smell, sound, etc.) and try to avoid them or forewarn them
- Concentrate on the child's strengths; allowing them to achieve and excel

- Teach older children to use public transportation, tech gadgets, and other helps in order to be more independent
- Teach them to respect themselves
- Teach them to love, honor, and obey the LORD

Parents of children with Asperger's can help their children by:

- Help your child practice appropriate reactions to common social situations at home so they can learn without feeling judged or on display.
- Teach your children the meaning of common phrases that aren't meant to be taken literally, since many children with Asperger's are quite literal. Example: Telling a child with Asperger's that he is silly will often get this type of response: "I'm not silly, I'm Max."

- Give your child a safety phrase— something to say that will alert you that they are feeling anxious and scared and unsure of how to respond or react.
- Prevent situations when possible rather than try to cure them after the fact.
- Plan ahead and keep your child informed of what they can expect. Surprises and the unexpected are NOT enjoyable to them.
- Don't argue with your child. Negotiate or end the conversation until both of you are better able to communicate rationally.
- Let them 'run with' the things that interest them and don't try to squelch their methods of imaginary play.

Whatever level of function your child has, remember this: They are precious in God's sight and are significant to His plan.

Chapter 8: Dealing With Special Neurological Needs

In an effort to encourage you to stay the course and keep things in their proper perspective, I want to offer you a list of tips and suggestions for dealing with the special needs of your child in a way that will benefit them and the rest of your family. Remember: Every child deserves to know, beyond a doubt, that the only reason you *need* to love them is because they are yours—that that's enough to merit your unconditional love.

Keeping that in mind, here are some things you can do to help your child with sensory processing disorder:

- Slow down. A lot of times children will be able to accept and enjoy new experiences if they are allowed to approach them at a slower pace.

- Give them space. Again, they need time to adjust to their surroundings and assess them in their own way.
- Keep things as visual as possible, as kids with sensory disorders are usually calmed by what they can see.
- Keep a bag full of items to distract your kids from sensory overload handy at ALL times.
- Be sensitive to their thoughts, feelings, and needs. Don't force things on them that aren't necessary.
- Introduce new sights, sounds, textures, and smells in a positive manner. Teach them to try something new, but let their response be the indicator of how far to take it.
- A therapy or specialized play group can be beneficial. Sometimes positive peer pressure works for the good of your child.

Children with auditory processing disorder:

- Should receive instructions in short, simple sentences. One step at a time.
- Should always be spoken to when facing them and when you are sure you have their attention.
- Keep things as visual as possible. Use chore charts, to-do lists, etc.
- Ask questions like: "Do you understand?" "Do you know what you are supposed to do?" "What did I just say to you?" Ask these questions in a loving, affirmative tone—not one that is condescending and degrading.
- Provide your child with simple puzzles, I-spy books, and toys that produce visible results.

Children with Tourette's and Epilepsy:

- Make sure your child takes their medication on schedule.
- Have regular medical checkups and evaluations.
- Make sure everyone in the family, teachers, and caregivers know what to do in the event of a seizure.
- Educate those who live and work with your child on the facts about Tourette's, Epilepsy, or other neurological disorder.
- Remember that the vast majority of children with Tourette's and Epilepsy have no mental or emotional disabilities. They are what society considers high-functioning children.
- Children with Epilepsy should always wear helmets when riding a bike or skating.

- Never allow an epileptic child to swim alone or be left alone in the tub. Older children should not be allowed to take a bath...showers only.
- Make sure your child has a medical alert bracelet or necklace on in the event they require emergency care and you are not with them. This will allow those around them to get the help your child needs.

REMEMBER: Awareness and knowledge are your child's two best allies when it comes to living with and thriving in spite of their special needs.

Bible Verses to Encourage You

You also, as living stones, are being built up a spiritual house, a holy priesthood, to offer up spiritual sacrifices acceptable to God through Jesus Christ. 1 Peter 2:5 (NKJV)

Be anxious for nothing, but in everything by prayer and supplication, with thanksgiving, let your requests be made known to God; and the peace of God, which surpasses all understanding, will guard your hearts and minds through Christ Jesus. ~Philippians 4:6-7

*Take heed that ye despise not one of these little ones; for I say unto you, that in heaven **their** angels do always behold the face of my Father which is in heaven. ~Matthew 18:10*

Chapter 9: Dealing with Genetic and Physical Special Needs

Among the most common physical and genetic problems facing parents of children with special needs include: cystic fibrosis, multiple sclerosis, cerebral palsy, downs syndrome, congenital birth defects of the vital organs or limbs, dyslexia, and muscular dystrophy.

There are of course, less common and even rare forms of these types of diseases and disorders including, dwarfism and SMA (spinal muscular atrophy)—to name just a few. And then there are those families dealing with special needs resulting from accidental injuries and problems resulting from the birth mother's abuse of drugs and alcohol.

No matter what the cause of the defect, disease, or injury, the fact remains that a child needs and deserves to enjoy the highest quality of life possible. Therefore, it is the wise and caring parent who makes the most of every opportunity and resource to help make that happen. You can be that parent when you:

- No matter what your child's special needs are, make sure everyone who lives with and spends time with your child on a regular basis knows what your child's condition is, what their needs are, has a working knowledge of how to meet those needs, and knows what to do in an emergency as well as how to do it.
- Make sure your child receives regular checkups and evaluations by their doctor and specialists.
- Make sure your child gets adequate rest, exercise (to the best of their ability), and social and intellectual stimulation and interaction.

- Make sure your child is eating a healthy and nutritious diet. Make this a family thing. For example: If your child is diabetic, don't make them feel deprived and different by keeping candy in the house for everyone else. Make it a special treat for everyone—even your diabetic on occasion.
- Be your child's advocate by taking whatever steps are necessary to ensure they receive the education they deserve and the assistance they need to reach their full potential.
- Do your homework. Stay up on the news concerning available resources for your child.

- Realize there are some things your child simply cannot do. When this happens you need to remember two things: 1) don't make your other children miss out on things. Let them enjoy the life they have been given. And 2) don't make a big deal out of it. Instead, focus on the things they *can* do and let them give those things 100%.

Children with Downs's Syndrome

- Embrace and enjoy their loving, affectionate nature.
- Encourage them to participate in social activities.
- Make sure they are receiving the best possible balance of mainstream classroom learning and classes targeted to meet their special needs. Downs kids are not dumb. They just need help learning how to express and use what they know.

- Parents of children with downs need to make exercise and healthy eating a priority to combat their tendency to be overweight and have heart problems.

Children with mobility needs

- Take your child for regular medical checkups and evaluations. Most mobility diseases and defects are progressive in nature; meaning they only get worse over time. You and your child need to know what is going on inside their body in order to meet their changing needs.
- Establish a regular routine for physical therapy. Movement of the right kind is essential for maintaining a quality of life for your child.
- Make sure your home is fully accessible to them. No child should feel unwelcome or in the way in their own home.

- Make sure your home is a safe place for your child. Loose rugs, exposed cords, and furniture that is unsteady can be hazardous.
- Equip your home in such a way that your child can grow into an independent young person. Make sure they can access the microwave and stovetop. Make sure the refrigerator opens in the direction necessary for them to be able to reach things easily. Make sure light switches are reachable. Lower the rods and shelves in their closet. Install a shower or tub to accommodate their needs with minimal or no assistance.

- Provide forms of exercise and entertainment they can enjoy at home: a swing set to accommodate their needs, a hot tub (ONLY with adult supervision), fuse ball, games with little or no physical movement required (trivia, etc.), audio books, and special instruments that will allow them to work the computer, and telephone.
- Take family outings that are wheelchair-friendly. Most state and national parks and sites are, as well as city parks, theaters, and amusement parks.

Children with genetic and other physical limitations

Genetic abnormalities can show themselves physically, mentally, or emotionally. The degree to which they show themselves also varies widely; ranging from things like dyslexia to an inability to speak or breathe without the assistance of a machine.

Because there are so many different forms or levels of special needs your child might have because of these things, it is important that you educate yourself as much as possible in regards to:

- The particulars of your child's needs and condition
- The resources available to you and your child
- What you can and cannot expect in the way of progression or digression
- What you should and shouldn't expect of your child
- How to properly care for your child
- How to help your child reach their full potential

When it's all is said and done, the most important thing you can remember as the parent of a special-needs child is that Jesus loves the little children - ALL the little children of the world – And that means Your Child too.

Bible Verses to Encourage You

Lo, children are a heritage of the Lord: and the fruit of the womb is His reward.
~Psalm 127:3

Behold the fowls of the air: for they sow not, neither do they reap, nor gather into barns; yet your heavenly Father feedeth them. Are ye not much better than they? ~Matthew 6:26

for I was hungry and you gave Me food; I was thirsty and you gave Me drink; I was a stranger and you took Me in; I was naked and you clothed Me; I was sick and you visited Me; I was in prison and you came to Me. "Then the righteous will answer Him, saying, 'Lord, when did we see You hungry and feed You, or thirsty and give You drink? When did we see You a stranger and take You in, or naked and clothe You? Or when did we see You sick, or in prison, and come to You?' And the King will answer and say to them, **'Assuredly, I say to you, inasmuch as you did it to one of the least of these My brethren, you did it to Me.'.** *~Matthew 25:35-40*

Chapter 10: Your Not-So-Secret Secret Thoughts

As the parent of a special-needs child you have thoughts and feelings parents of other kids don't have. You think:

- Why my child? Why don't they get to run and play? Why can't they enjoy something as simple as licking an ice cream cone or sloshing through a mud puddle in their bare feet? Why do they have to be the one kids make fun of and shy away from?
- Why doesn't God answer my prayers to heal my child? He healed all those other people in the Bible?
- If I hear the term 'short bus', 'retard', or 'freak' one more time I'm going to explode all over whoever says it.

- I just wish I could have one day that was the kind of normal most people have.
- I know they say it's not my fault, but…but…is it…maybe?

And yes, some of you have even thought:

- If we wouldn't have had this to deal with, our marriage would have survived.
- It's not fair to my other children for me to have to devote so much of myself to their sibling.
- My husband or wife and I are never going to know what it's like to be just the two of us.
- What's going to happen to him/her when we can no longer take care of him/her? Who will take over?
- I'm so tired I don't know if I can do this again tomorrow.

You are only human, so it is natural for you to become weary, worried, and worn down. But the great news is—the news you *have to hold tight to*—is that you don't have to remain weary, worried, and worn down. God the Father, Jesus the Son, and the Holy Spirit are here to help. They are here to take these things from you and replace them with rest, peace, and hope.

As we close out our 'time' together, I want to leave you with some final words of encouragement from the scripture. My prayer is that these words will inspire you to be thankful for and mindful of the fact that you have been chosen by God to care for and rise up one of his extra-special children.

God bless you abundantly!

Bible Verses to Encourage You

Casting down arguments and every high thing that exalts itself against the knowledge of God, bringing every thought into captivity to the obedience of Christ; ~2 Corinthians 10:5

Finally, brethren, whatever things are true, whatever things are noble, whatever things are just, whatever things are pure, whatever things are lovely, whatever things are of good report, if there is any virtue and if there is anything praiseworthy—meditate on these things. ~Philippians 4:8

*I beseech you therefore, brethren, by the mercies of God, that you present your bodies a living sacrifice, holy, acceptable to God, which is your reasonable service. And do not be conformed to this world, but be transformed by the renewing of your mind, that you may prove what is that good and acceptable and perfect will of God.
~Romans 12:1-2*

WISDOM FROM YOUR ELDERS

Learning From Your Parents, Grandparents, and the Older People in Your Church

By: Patrick Baldwin

Introduction

Proverbs 1:8 says, *"My son, hear the instruction of thy father, and forsake not the law of thy mother...."* How many times have you said that to your kids? How many times did you *hear* that as a kid? Okay, so maybe not those exact words, but the message was the same: "Listen to me." "Do what I tell you." Or possibly even, "Are you pickin' up what I'm puttin' down?"

The words used isn't all that important. What *is* important, however, is that the message be both sent and received. Equally important is that the message be transmitted with consistency and regularity—by our attitudes, words, and actions.

This book is designed with the young person in mind. However, this book is also for parents, grandparents, and everyone else who has a regular connection with a child or teenager. Its purpose is to a) remind you that it is your job to instill wisdom and common sense into the hearts and minds of the generation coming after you b) give you practical ways to accomplish this task and c) help you do your job in such a way that it inspires and prepares the children and young people in your life to be ready to do the same...someday.

My prayer is that you will live the words in this book by applying them to your life in order to raise up a generation of young people who will be ready to:

- Lead the Church in sound doctrine and with the compassion of Jesus
- Establish Godly families
- Live lives based on solid faith and integrity

I know that sounds like a monumental-sized task. But it's not. All it really requires is for you to make a personal investment into the lives of the children and young people you know and love. So yes, while it *sounds* like a monumental-sized task, it's not. But it *does* have monumental-sized rewards.

Chapter 1: Foundations of Relationships

We're going to start things off by simply looking at a number of verses in the Bible that address cross-generational relationships and 'discuss' how they apply to the world we live in today.

WARNING: some of the verses we are getting ready to look at are going to broach subjects like respect, honoring traditions, making changes, and embracing our roles. In other words, some of you are about to get a little uncomfortable. Or as my grandma would say, you're about to get your toes stepped on. But please don't let that keep you from doing your job the way God intends for you to. Besides, what's a little 'pain' when you know you will reap the rewards of your labor *and* be able to go to bed at night knowing you are making an impact for the kingdom of God?

So are you ready? Let's get started….

*Children's children are the crown of old men;
and the glory of children are their fathers.*
~Proverbs 17:6

This verse paints a beautiful picture of the unity God intends us to have across the generations. It joins three generations together in a circle—one that is meant to be unbroken.

First let's look at the relationship between children and their grandparents (children's children). The Hebrew word for crown means to hold a place of honor or to be honorable. The responsibility here lies with the children's children (the youngest generation). They are to live honorable lives that reflect back on their grandparents in a positive way. In today's language, we would simply say, "They do us proud."

The last part of the verse places the burden of responsibility on the parents (the middle generation). They are to bring glory to their children—to be someone their children can count on…depend on…look up to.

Everyone has ownership in the relationship. Everyone invests. Everyone benefits.

One generation shall praise thy works to another, and shall declare thy mighty acts.
~Psalm 145:4

The message here is that each generation has a responsibility to bring their children and grandchildren up to know God. Not just know about him, but *know* Him.

Judges 2:10-11 is both a perfect and tragic example of what happens when we don't live according to this verse. Look at what happens…

After that whole generation had been gathered to their ancestors, another generation grew up who knew neither the Lord nor what He had done for Israel. Then the Israelites did evil in the eyes of the Lord and served the Baals.

People, the generation that was 'gathered' was the generation that crossed the Red Sea as children. They were the generation of people who ate the manna provided by God. They were the generation of people who grew up seeing God's amazing love as well as His anger displayed in some of the most amazing ways recorded in the Bible. So why, oh why, didn't they tell their children?

Why did they allow the next generation to grow up without knowing how and why they were able to live in the land "flowing with milk and honey"?

We'll never know the answer to that question. We do, however, know what happened because they failed to live out this verse. Israel lost its place of honor in God's heart and mind. They had their inheritance ripped from them and were handed over to the Godless.

Don't do this to your kids. Don't do this to your grandkids and to future generations. Set an example, teach with words and actions the value and essentiality of knowing God in a real and personal way.

Only take heed to thyself, and keep thy soul diligently, lest thou forget the things which thine eyes have seen, and lest they depart from thy heart all the days of thy life: but teach them thy sons, and thy sons' sons; ~Deuteronomy 4:9

This verse is another reminder—a warning even, against neglecting your spiritual wellbeing.

The first part of the verse speaks of the importance of being diligent in pursuing a relationship with God for *your* sake. You need to guard *your* heart and mind against apathy and sin so that *you* can experience the blessed life God created you to have.

Moses was essentially saying, "Pay attention to what I am about to say and *obey...live by* the laws I am about to give you because they are from the LORD."

The second half of the verse is the multi-generational part. We are told to teach our sons and daughters these things. And just in case you've already forgotten 'these things'—'these things' being the laws and instructions from God given through Moses.

The laws and instructions from God referenced here are not limited to 'just' matters of faith and spirituality. It is a lot more than that. The 'these things' Moses was talking about was the entire Law (of Moses, as it is commonly called) that God set in place for the people to live by. So while faith and matters of spirituality should be the foundation upon which everything else is taught, it isn't the only thing one generation is responsible for passing down to the next.

Hear, O Israel: The Lord our God is one Lord: And thou shalt love the Lord thy God with all thine heart, and with all thy soul, and with all thy might. And these words, which I command thee this day, shall be in thine heart: And thou shalt teach them diligently unto thy children, and shalt talk of them when thou sittest in thine house, and when thou walkest by the way, and when thou liest down, and when thou risest up. And thou shalt bind them for a sign upon thine hand, and they shall be as frontlets between thine eyes. And thou shalt write them upon the posts of thy house, and on thy gates.
~Deuteronomy 6:4-9

This is one of my favorite passages of scripture because it is so explicit and literal. There's no wiggle-room for misconstruing what God wants. No, what God *expects* of parents and grandparents. So let's take a few minutes to pick this verse apart and see what it is telling us to do.

Love the LORD thy God with all thine heart, and with all thy soul, and with all they might. Love the LORD with *everything* you've got. And do it twenty-four/seven.

...teach them diligently unto thy children…. The word diligent means to be thorough, persistent, conscientious, deliberate, consistent, and attentive. There's nothing happenstance or random about it. In order for this to happen, though, YOU have to be in sync with God. YOU have to be living what you speak.

The next few phrases in this passage instruct us to **talk about God's commands** when we are **sitting, walking, as we put our children to bed at night,** and **when we get up to start a new day.** Here again this is a strong and indisputable indication that God intends our teaching to come from *who we are* not *what we do.* It's lifestyle vs. compliance.

Example: Parents who pray with their children, pray for their children, worship and serve the LORD with their children in public, *and* who operate their marriage and home on the same principles are living obediently to God and to this passage of scripture. Parents who pray at mealtimes, go to church occasionally, or who are faithful attenders but the atmosphere of their home and their business dealings would indicate otherwise are not living up to God's expectations.

Putting these things on your hand and on the 'frontlets' between your eyes—now that's something you don't hear every day. These statements are referring to the common cultural practices of the day in regards to what the people wore. Translating it into something we can relate to, however, isn't difficult. Basically what God is saying here is that our appearance should reflect our relationship with God. We should teach our children to dress appropriately and to take care of their bodies.

We will discuss this subject more in depth later on, but for now, let's just say that while it isn't fair or even right to judge a book by its cover, our appearance does say something about us, so we need to teach our children to make sure they always send the right message—that they are a child of God.

Writing 'these things' on the posts and gates of our houses is simply God's way of telling us to make God's Word the foundation of our home. Fill your home with visible and tangible reminders of God's Word. But don't just throw a few magnets on the fridge, toss a pillow on the couch with a scripture verse on it, and buy a 'verse of the day' calendar every year. LIVE IT!

I have to tell you about an incident I witnessed in a store one day that is the perfect example of someone who surely had 'these things' written on the posts and gates of his home.

I was in a home décor store looking for something when I walked by a man talking to one of the store clerks. In his hand he had a wooden plaque with a scripture verse painted on it. I didn't think much of it, but because I was looking at some items directly across from them, I couldn't help but hear their conversation. It went like this…

Man: "I don't mean to be rude and I'm not saying this is your fault, but you really should sell this item like this." (hold the plaque out toward the clerk.

Clerk: "Why not?"

Man: "Well, because it's wrong."

The man then began to read: "In their hearts humans plan their course, but the Lord establishes their steps."

Clerk: "What's wrong with that? I think it's nice. It just reminds people who believe in God to have faith in him."

Man: "Oh, I know. And I'm all for that. I'm a preacher."

Confused clerk: "So then why are you telling me it's wrong?"

Man: "Look at the bottom. It says this verse is Psalm 19:16. It's not. There isn't even such a thing as Psalm 19:16 and the verse is Proverbs 16:9. "

Clerk: "Oh. Ummm..."

Man: "Like I said, I'm not trying to be rude and I know you had nothing to do with it. I'm just saying it's misleading. Or in my business," he laughed, "false advertising."

Like I said, this guy had 'these things' on his posts and his gates. And no, it wasn't just because he was a preacher. It was because he knows the Word of God.

This isn't to say grandparents and parents have to memorize the Bible or know it from cover to cover. But remember…you cannot live and you cannot teach what you do not know. So ready, study, live, and teach God's Word to your children.

That the aged men be sober, grave, temperate, sound in faith, in charity, in patience. Young men likewise exhort to be sober minded. ~Titus 2:2 and 6

These verses are part of Paul's letter to Titus on how to teach and train the Christians in Crete. There are two things I really like about these verses. The first is that they clearly state the need and expectation for intentional mentorship by the older mean of the church to the younger men in the church. The fact that relationships are to be a part of this mentorship cannot be overlooked or dismissed. To exhort means to urge, encourage, and counsel (advise). These things cannot happen without being relational.

The second thing that sticks out to me is that these verses aren't limited to Biblical teaching.

They don't let the older men off by telling them to make sure the younger men know how to pray in public, pass the communion trays correctly, and say a few 'amen's' at the right time. No, exhorting the young men to be charitable, patient, temperate, sober-minded, and faithful requires a lot more time and energy than could be given during a church service. Times haven't changed in this regard—not even since way back then.

Teaching the next generation of men to be charitable requires the old and the young to work together to know who is in need, what their needs are, and then actively participate in meeting those needs.

Patience—that's a tricky one, because patience is something a person has to do themselves. No one can give it to you or force it upon you. A person can, however, learn what patience looks like and its value on their relationships and life in general by seeing it in someone else.

So by taking on challenges together (the old and the young) that require patience, and by simply sharing life stories and experiences in how exhibiting patience has served them well, the younger generation can learn from the older generation.

To be temperate and sober-minded doesn't sound like much fun, does it? It kind of reminds me of the old bachelor that lived at the end of our road. He never waved or smiled when we drove by. The only person that ever came to see him was his sister. He was, quite honestly, an old grouch. But that's not what it means—not at all.

To be temperate and sober-minded means to be **calm, self-controlled, composed, peaceable, measured, sensible, and alert.**

Not a bad list of character traits, right? But let's be realistic. How many calm, composed, self-controlled, and sensible twenty-one year-old men do you know?

I think every single guy out there over the age of forty would have to admit that their twenty-something self didn't always handle things the way they should have been handled. But here's the thing—unless the twenty-something young man has a dad, grandpa, and/or other older men to look to, listen to, and learn from, he is never going to fully outgrow his impetuousness. He's never going to fully learn how to or the merits of:

- Thinking before he speaks
- Knowing when he needs to not speak at all
- Extending grace
- Knowing what actually is (and isn't) important
- Responding rather than reacting
- Empathy, sympathy, and compassion
- Being aware of his surroundings in order to keep himself and his family safe, to not be taken advantage of, and to know what is and isn't spiritually beneficial and uplifting

- Making sound judgements and decisions based on fact and Godly principles vs. emotions and peer pressure

In other words, young men need dads, grandpas, and other mentors to help them grow up in the LORD.

The aged women likewise, that they be in behaviour as becometh holiness, not false accusers, not given to much wine, teachers of good things; That they may teach the young women to be sober, to love their husbands, to love their children, to be discreet, chaste, keepers at home, good, obedient to their own husbands, that the word of God be not blasphemed. ~Titus 2:3-5

Paul didn't want anyone to be left out. So along with the verses we just looked at regarding the relationships in (and out of) the church between men of different generations, he addresses what the older women need to be teaching the younger women.

Women, too, are to be sober-minded. But when you are trying to juggle a baby, making sure your second-grader knows their spelling words, getting the house ready for company, taking your ten year-old to soccer practice, and trying to find time to get your Bible study lesson done...in case you actually get to go this week.... It's not easy to stay calm or respond instead of letting those knee-jerk reactions spew out. And showing mercy by dropping off a lunch box to the child who forgot their lunch for the third day this month—well, it's just not there. Not without the encouragement of someone who has been-there-done-that, anyway.

If younger women don't have older women to encourage them and remind them that this too, really will pass, they younger women tend to close ranks, talk (gripe) among themselves, and develop a don't-mess-with-me-or-I'll-make-your-life-miserable attitude. Either that or one that gives up on seeing the joy and immeasurable value of her job and as a result, ends up bitter, resentful, anxious, and depressed.

Not a pretty picture is it? But it is a picture that never has to be seen if women will embrace the instructions of God's Word by taking the time to invest themselves into the lives of their younger peers.

Older Godly women can teach younger women to slow down and enjoy their children. They can teach them that a healthy *marriage* is something you never stop working at and that the kind of love that takes a marriage through a lifetime is something you *do*—not something you get or have.

These verses also place the responsibility on the older women to teach the younger women about things like modesty, purity, submission to their husbands, and being a homemaker. As I look at this list I realize most of these things are considered old-fashioned and non-issues in today's society. And if you are one of those people who feel this way, let me ask you this: How's that working for you? How's that working for society?

Excuses like:

- They (the younger girls/women) won't listen to me
- They (the older women) don't understand what it's like today
- Those rules are out of date
- That was for then—not for now
- I'm not a slave—I'm a wife

Anything along these lines simply don't let you off the hook. Hebrews 13:8 tells us that Jesus Christ is the same yesterday, today, and forever. He doesn't change. Neither do his expectations and commands—even if we think they should.

When Christian women from different generations join hearts and minds, life becomes better for everyone involved. God is glorified. The Church is strengthened and enriched. Homes are happier and healthier. Marriages thrive and last a lifetime. Children feel secure, confident, and know what it means to be loved unconditionally. In short, everyone wins.

When I call to remembrance the unfeigned faith that is in thee, which dwelt first in thy grandmother Lois, and thy mother Eunice; and I am persuaded that is in thee also. ~2 Timothy 1:5

This verse is yet another reminder to parents and grandparents that it is OUR responsibility to raise our children and grandchildren to know Jesus as their Savior in a personal way. It is a reminder to us that children truly do learn what they live.

So teach us to number our days, that we may apply our hearts unto wisdom. ~Psalm 90:12

And finally...in all of our teaching (and I am speaking here to the older generations), we cannot forget that we also need to keep growing and learning.

I was talking to a friend of mine about the fact that I was going to write this book. She then shared with me how blessed she had been in her years as a young wife and mother to be part of a small congregation that included a number of women old enough to be her mom and her grandma. In fact, she said, "One of them was my own grandma."

She went on to tell me how these women ministered to her and to one another. "I knew my entire family could count on being loved and cared for by these women. And not just at church. Phone calls throughout the week, birthday cards, hugs and kisses when we ran into each other in the store, fellowship in their homes…we had relationships. And the women who were what she called the middle generation—older than her, but younger than her grandma and some of the others—they looked up to the older women as much as I did. And they were ministered to in the same way I was."

Isn't that beautiful? That's what Paul was talking about in his letter to Titus. That's what God was telling the Israelites. That's what the Psalmist and Solomon were talking about. The Bible is filled with words of instruction on investing ourselves into the lives of those younger than us. So let's do it—let's be obedient to God's Word and raise up a generation of young people ready to carry on the work of the Church God's way.

Chapter 2: Benefits for Young People

What benefits are there for young people to develop deep relationships with their elders?

The benefits of spending time with your elders are both countless and priceless. Here are just a few (in no particular order of importance):

Respect

- The student cannot help but be humbled by the wisdom that comes from life-experiences and the teacher's appreciation and understanding of the need to be recognized as an adult rather than a child is renewed.

Work Ethic

- Older people are generally more industrious because they had to be and it was a habit they never let go of. Younger people need to understand that things haven't always been instant, pre-packaged, or ready-to-wear.

- They also need to know how to adjust in case they find themselves in a position of not having the luxury of everything at their fingertips.

Life-Skills

- I could go on and on about the negative effects of not cooking from scratch, making something from start to finish, and being self-sufficient when it comes to simple house maintenance, car work, and so on. But I won't. Instead, I'll just say that when older men and women teach their younger peers how to do these things, the younger men and women experience a sense of accomplishment not able to be found anywhere else.

Tenacity

- Giving up wasn't an option back then and the current generation needs to know it shouldn't be an option now.

- You don't quit a job just because you don't like it or someone hurts your feelings. You don't quit on your spouse just because you don't agree on how things should be done, you don't like your in-laws, or you don't feel validated and fulfilled. You don't quit trying to overcome bad spending habits, addictions, or a sinful lifestyles because it's too hard or it doesn't make you feel good. Older people know that there really is light at the end of those tunnels. So in spending time with them, younger people learn to keep looking for that light.

Wisdom

- Wisdom must generally come with age. Not always, mind you, but when God is in the equation, it is pretty much a sure thing. I know there are just some things we have to learn for ourselves—some mistakes we have to make for ourselves.

- But younger people can save themselves a lot of trouble, expense, and heartache by learning from those who have been-there-done-that.

Active Faith

- Faith in action can and should be seen in people of all ages. But when younger people are able to see active faith in older people, they are exposed to the aspect of longevity. Parents, grandparents, and older people in the church are living testimonies of the blessings that come from living a life of faith. Once more, they can offer hope and encouragement in times of doubt. They can offer proof that the grief of losing a loved one does turn to sweet memories and hope for an eternal reunion. They can offer advice on how to hear and see God working in the lives of those that seek Him.

Unconditional Love

- By the time you get to the age where you are considered older or elderly, if you know God, you know His love is unconditional. Why else would you still be able to feel and experience that love, right? If it wasn't unconditional, you would have been gone a long time ago. Young people need to know this. They need to know that there is almost nothing God won't or can't forgive when we come to Him in true repentance. This is something young people can't really learn from their peers, because their peers are experiencing the very same doubts. By reaching across the generations, older people provide tangible proof that no one is too much of a mess for Jesus.

Good Stewardship

- Older people know what it means to go without. They know full-well we don't need half of what we think we do. They know how to make a dollar stretch. They know how to improvise, re-purpose, and to live a more simplified and less stressful lifestyle. They don't have to have the newest and best and they know why you (younger people) don't have to have those things, either. In listening to their stories and watching their ways, younger people can learn to be less materialistic. They can learn to recognize and appreciate what really matters in life. They come to learn that *"a parent's presence is far more important to a child than their presents"*.

Patience

- Again, this is just one of those things learned over time and experience. But when younger people hear someone older saying, "Be patient. It will all work out the way it's supposed to." Or, "Wait on God's timing and remember that God's timing is always perfect." it has a soothing and reassuring effect. It's like faith fertilizer.

Faith fertilizer—I like that, don't you? In fact, if I had to sum up the content of this chapter, this is what I would say: Younger generations of Christians should take every opportunity to be friends with, fellowship with, serve with, and minister with (and to) their parents, grandparents, and the older people in their church. Why? Because in doing so, they get regular applications of faith (and life) fertilizer; causing them to grow and thrive spiritually and emotionally in the LORD and in their relationships with others.

Yes, that's it—that's what building relationships can do for young people.

Chapter 3: Benefits for Older People

Often times we think of these relationships as being one-sided in regards to their benefits. It's the younger people who learn new skills. It's the younger people who receive the attention. It's the younger people who are spared trouble and pain by learning from the mistakes of others.

The truth of the matter, however, is that parents, grandparents, and other adults have just as much to gain (and learn) from these relationships as the younger people do.

I think the number-one benefit is that the older person is fulfilling their role in scripture. They are being obedient to God. They are being teachers, disciple-makers, mentors, evangelists, parents, role models….Christians.

The next benefit I see is that of accountability.
When I think of the accountability factor I think about the words of Hebrews 13:7: *Remember your leaders, who spoke the word of God to you. Consider the outcome of their way of life and imitate their faith. (NIV)*

You are being watched, mimicked and looked up to. And that, my friend, is powerful. Your words, actions, and attitudes are shaping those of the children and young adults in your sphere of influence. Knowing you have this kind of influence should keep you on your toes. No, you aren't perfect and you shouldn't claim to be. But knowing you are helping to shape and form the opinions and attitudes of others in regards to genuine Christianity should cause you to examine yourself more closely.

Parents, grandparents, and other adults who take the time to invest themselves into the lives of the young people they know and love, also set themselves up to receive the following

- Patience. Spending time with younger people 'forces' older generations to slow down to explain why. Explain why again…and possibly even again. Older adults are also reminded that their younger counterparts don't always know how to use tools or perform household tasks; requiring them to teach a young person how.

- Hope. This goes back to my number one benefit—fulfilling their role in scripture. Relationships between generations bring a sense of hope for the future of the Church to older people. When older people *know* they have done their best to teach, equip, and disciple the children and young people in sound doctrine and to be the hands, feet, eyes, and ears of Jesus, they don't have to worry about what is going to happen to the future generation. They know it is in good hands.

- Stimulation. Let's face it—parents, and especially grandparents, are sometimes guilty of being set in their ways. Fostering relationships with the younger generation keeps you on your toes. You stay 'in the know' (at least somewhat) on pop culture. You see things from a younger perspective. You feel younger (in an appropriate way). You consider and sometimes adopt a different mindset than what you previously had.

- Appreciation and respect for others. Listening to and caring about the thoughts and opinions of young people teaches you to respect them. You get an up-close and personal view of their intellect, compassion, and their desire to leave a positive imprint on society.

- Friendship. You can never have too many of those, can you?

- A stronger sense of purpose and usefulness. Relationships with people from different generations will allow you to share your knowledge, wisdom, skills, talents, and passions with others. You feel needed. Wanted. Useful.

Sharing life with people outside your generational peer group is a win-win situation for everyone involved. Don't you agree?

Chapter 4: Fostering Strong Relationships

Now that you have been reminded of why your relationships should reach across the generations, let's get down to the nuts and bolts of how to go about getting the job done.

What follows is a list of things you can do on the home front to form a stronger bond with the young people in your life. Just remember to be sincere. No one wants to feel like a charity case or an assignment. Be flexible and be yourself. Don't have unrealistic expectations. Give your children the freedom to be themselves too. Give the relationship to God and enjoy the blessings He sends because of it.

Tell stories. Sharing stories about your life when you were their age is a great way to connect. It also allows you to insert messages like "If I'd only known then what I know now" and "I sure wish I wouldn't have done that" all without sounding judgmental or 'preachy'.

Cook together. It doesn't have to be cooking. It can be any hobby or similar task as long as it allows you to accomplish something together. These types of activities are great for casual conversation and teachable moments. Don't let them get away from you.

Work together. Cleaning the garage, servicing the car, yard work-whatever needs to be done. Working together allows you to teach important life-skills and prepare them for when they are out on their own.

Teach a skill or hobby. Passing on the gift of a particular skill or hobby to the next generation has proven to be one of the best ways to solidify relationships with people of different generations. It's a passing of the torch kind of thing.

Volunteer. Did you know that schools would rather have grandparent-age volunteers than any other age group? There are numerous reasons why, but their wisdom, their sense of responsibility, and the students' positive response and interaction with them are at the top or the list. Teenagers like spending time with older grandparent-type people because they aren't always in a hurry to get to or from work or too busy to just sit and hang out and listen. Students also respond to this age group's storytelling method of advice giving better than they do their parents' more direct approach.

Chaperone events. You can build positive relationships with the teenagers in your life just by being present. When chaperoning events either at church, school, or in the community, you don't have to say much. Your presence sends the message that you are about them— that you want them to have a safe, fun, and wholesome environment to be a teenager. Your presence also says that you think they are worth your time and energy.

Cheer them on. Showing up for games, recitals, performances, meets, matches, etc. sends the message that you care. You are proud. You support them. You believe in them. Don't think they don't notice when you are there...and when you aren't. And don't think that just because they don't shower you with hugs and kisses they aren't glad to see you. They are.

Play together. Introduce them to the games and activities you played when you were their age and ask them to teach you how to play something they enjoy playing.

Pray for the children in your life. There is no greater gift you can give the teenagers in your life than to cover them with prayer.

Talk to the children in your life. Talking to your teenagers about current events, what's going on at school, what's going on with friends, and about what's going on in your life, as well. Don't confuse talking with inquisition. Talking is conversation *between* the two of you.

Listen to the children in your life. Listening is at least as important as talking. Listen to what they have to say. Ask them how they feel about things, what they think about things, and what their goals are. Listen not only to their words, but their moods and their feelings.

Give them ownership in their family's history. Telling stories about past generations, letting them know where their family came from, and making sure they understand the significance of family heirlooms is a great way to stay connected with the teens in your family. They need to know the personal and emotional ties to the pretty bowl they were never allowed to touch or to the necklace they know will "Someday be yours."

Ask their opinion and advice. Teenagers are really caught in a holding pattern. They aren't children, but they aren't adults, either. This often leaves them feeling disrespected and undervalued. You can solve this by asking their opinion and advice on things.

They are far more tech-savvy than you'll ever be, so ask for their help. You'll both benefit. Ask their opinions on current events and politics. If their mindset seems to be more world-focused than God-focused, you can then use the opportunity to discuss the matter in a calm, rational manner—and help them see things from a spiritual perspective. Ask them what they prefer to have for dinner one or two nights a week. Ask them if they would like to help plan (or be in charge of planning) the family's next outing or plans for their birthday. Ask them about…well, you get the point.

Include them in conversations and some decision-making processes. Yes, I know there are some things kids (even teenagers) don't need to weigh in on. But when it comes to things like where to vacation, whether or not to relocate, bringing Grandma to live with you, or how to tighten up the family's budget, allowing your teenager to weigh in isn't a bad idea.

Allowing them to express their thoughts and feelings gives them a sense of ownership in the family. It validates their sense of self-worth and the fact that you respect them. They do, however, need to understand that just because they are allowed to weigh in doesn't mean things will always go their way. This needs to be understood from the onset in order to avoid problems. But when handled properly, allowing them to be part of these processes helps build a more positive relationship between a teenager and his/her parents and grandparents.

See, that's not so hard, is it? Now get out there and start getting to know your teenagers better than you ever thought possible!

Chapter 5: Relationships in the Church

Below you will find a list of practical ways to build solid and lasting relationships between the teenagers and older people in the church.

Numerous youth in my life would tell you just how much of an impact these relationships have had on their lives. They would also tell you that there was nothing orchestrated or prefabricated about these relationships. They happened as a result of one or more of the following:

Teach. Who better to teach a group of teenagers than someone who has the knowledge and spiritual wisdom you have? Teaching sound doctrine and the message of the Gospel gives you the peace of mind that the young people of your church are being equipped to lead in the future.

Worship together. God intends the church to be a family. We can't really be a family, though, if we don't come together to worship God, the father of our family. Worshipping together creates a bond of unity with those around you no matter how old or young you are.

Volunteer. You cannot have relationships with people you don't know. Volunteer to chaperone youth group events. Volunteer to host them in your home for Bible study or for a special event. Volunteer to share your testimony with the teens during their weekly meeting. Volunteer to help plan and organize events for them.

Give. Donate your time and talents to provide food for their events. Remember—teenagers LOVE to eat. Donate funds so that teens that couldn't otherwise do so, can go to church camp, on a mission trip, or other such event.

Work together. Make sure your church includes the teenagers for church work days. Not only does it allow you to spend time together, but it gives the older people the chance to teach the younger people important skills.

Serve together. Don't exclude teenagers from service projects in the church. Serve together. Remember...the church is a family.

Pray for the teens in your church. This one needs no explanation. Just do it. And mention them by name. Additionally, when you take the time to get to know them, you will know what you need to be praying about.

Fellowship together. Again, don't exclude teenagers from times of fellowship with the adults by always having segregated events.

Use the teens in your church. Hire the teens in your church to mow your lawn, clean out your attic or basement, paint your fence, pet sit, etc... Having them in your home allows you to get to know one another and allows you to share Jesus in simple, yet meaningful ways.

Invest in their lives outside of church. Notice when their accomplishments are mentioned in the paper and compliment them for their achievements. Send them birthday cards. Talk to them at church. Ask them about school. Offer to tutor them or teach them a skill. Attend their extra-curricular activities.

Train them. Too often older people complain that the future of their local congregation is in jeopardy because of a lack of spiritual maturity in the hearts of the young people. Don't be one of those people. Instead, train up the teenagers in your church so that they will be thoroughly equipped for every good work (2 Timothy 3:16-17).

Give them responsibility. There's nothing a teenager hates more than being treated like a little kid. So don't. Give them appropriate responsibilities in the church. Let them be part of the praise team. Lead music. Offer public prayer. Serve communion. Work in the nursery. Teach or assist teaching younger children. Play on church-league sports teams. Greet people. Read the scripture publically. You get the picture.

Building relationships across the generations really isn't all that hard to do. Just like making friends among your same-age peers, all it takes is your heart, your time and a dose of effort.

Chapter 6: A Sense of Responsibility

Among the things older people often fault the younger generations for is their lack of responsibility. They (older people) complain that their children and/or grandchildren don't have the same sense of responsibility they were raised with—that they don't know what it means to be held accountable for their actions.

I'm not going to argue against this point of view, because society and statistics prove that teenagers and young adults *are* less responsible than their parents and especially, their grandparents. But now I'm going to tell you something you won't want to hear: We (as in older adults) don't have anyone but ourselves to blame.

Over the past several decades parents have had the mindset that they needed to make things easier for their kids than they had it.

While that sounds nice in theory, in reality, it has created a generation or two of young people that neither know nor appreciate the sense of self-worth and accomplishment that comes with being responsible. That's right—we did it to them and to ourselves.

What to do? Fix it, that's what! Or at least, do our best to try—and here's how...

Set a good example by being responsible yourself.

Don't wait until your teenagers become teenagers to teach them how to be responsible. Okay, so that's the ideal situation, but if that ship has sailed, don't think it's too late. It might require more effort and patience on your part, but both you and your teens will be better for it.

Provide opportunities for your teens to practice and exhibit responsibility. This means that once you give them a task to do or mission to accomplish, don't rescue them. Don't intervene and 'fix' things. Let them (require them) to complete the task or mission all on their own.

Allow them to experience both the rewards and the consequences of their actions. Responsibility isn't just about paying the consequences for the mistakes or poor choices you make. The positive aspects of responsibility are equally important—reaping the rewards of a job well done. Allowing teenagers to experience both is an important life lesson in decision making and for learning that they have the power to decide the direction their life takes.

Have realistic expectations for your teenager and expect them to live up to those expectations.

As I was typing that sentence I was thinking of Queen Esther. We don't know for sure how old Esther was when her cousin/father Mordecai, insisted that she step up and take responsibility for the safety of her people. But history and cultural practices of the day tell us she was a virgin; indicating she was still very young—most likely in her very early teens—when she went to live in the palace and ultimately become the queen of the Persian Empire.

Mordecai's expectations didn't come out of nowhere or even out of desperation. He knew Esther was capable of carrying out the mission because he had raised her to be responsible. Yes, she needed a little encouragement and gentle prodding, but he knew she could do it **because he had taught her the hows and whys of responsibility.**

Can you say the same?

Chapter 7: Patience

I know, I know—patience isn't something you pray for, because the only way to get it is to have to use it. It's one of those 'practice makes perfect' kind of things. Patience is also something we all need in abundance; making it an essential character trait we need to help our teenagers develop.

Passing on the quality of patience is a lot like passing on any other character trait. It happens best when we show them how, give them opportunities to practice it, and expect them to exhibit it.

In teaching these things to your teenager, it is also important to make sure they understand what patience really is. The dictionary defines patience in the following way:

PATIENCE: the capacity to accept or tolerate delay, trouble, or suffering without getting angry or upset

Patience is also, and ultimately, learning to trust in God's timing and His will for our lives. Teaching your teen to be patient from this perspective is the perfect opportunity to help them grow their faith and grow in their knowledge of the scriptures.

David and Jesse are an excellent example of what this 'looks like'. David was just a boy when Samuel the High Priest came to Jesse; telling him God had chosen one of his sons to be the next king of Israel. There was one condition though—he wouldn't take the throne for quite some time. David would be king, but he would need to be patient and wait for God's timing.

David had no problem with that. In fact, in reading the last several chapters of the book of First Samuel, you will see that David even resisted getting Saul out of the picture on more than one occasion.

David's ability to wait patiently didn't just happen. It was the result of being brought up to know that God's timing and authority is perfect and worthy of our complete trust.

Some practical ways to help teach your teen to be more patient include:

- Model patience. I know I've already said that, but it's worth repeating.
- Work together on a project that requires patience. Landscaping, painting a room in your house, refinishing a piece of furniture, fishing, hunting, or playing board games like "Monopoly", "Candy Land" or "Scrabble", and gardening are all good patience-builders.
- Orchestrate delays that will require your teens to wait. Arrive early to an event. Serve dinner a bit later than usual. Tell them they have to wait until their birthday or Christmas to get their phone upgrade or something similar they want.

- Don't allow them to experience 'instant gratification' too often. Make them wait until they have earned the extra money they need to buy that certain pair of shoes or the jeans they 'have to have' because everyone else has a pair. Don't buy or serve fast-food or instant anything. Cook...from scratch.

In teaching your teens what patience *is,* you also need to be sure you teach them what patience is *not.* Patience is NOT:

- Allowing others to take advantage of you.
- Allowing people to habitually mistreat you, abuse the privileges of friendship, or disrespect you by ignoring your needs.
- Procrastination.
- Allowing others to consistently procrastinate at your expense.

How well are you doing in passing on the trait of patience?

Chapter 8: Faith

Previously I made mention of Hebrews 13:7 which says, "Remember your leaders, who spoke the word of God to you. Consider the outcome of their way of life and imitate their faith." (NIV) This verse is obviously speaking to the younger generations, i.e. young people in this instance, but at the heart of this verse is a message we 'leaders' must not miss. It is the message that leaders are to:

- Speak the Word of God to the younger generations
- Live a life of faith that is worthy of being imitated
- Serve as spiritual mentors to the younger generation by setting an example in how you worship, serve others, fellowship, and grow in your knowledge of the Word

Speaking the Word of God to the younger generations is essential for passing on and instilling in them the need and desire for a strong faith.

After all, a person really can't put your faith in something you know little or nothing about. We can't expect the young people in our lives to live according to the Word if they don't know what that word is. What's more, we cannot and should not expect them to read, understand, and discern it all on their own. They need the wisdom and understanding that comes from studying over a period of time, aka age.

Jonah spoke God's message to the people of Nineveh. Peter spoke the message of the Gospel to countless people around him. Paul also took the Gospel to the known world of his day; preaching the message of salvation through Jesus. And of course Jesus himself spoke the message of truth to all He encountered.

Your way of life in 'church talk' is "your Christian walk". Are you setting a good example with your attitude? Your actions? Your speech?

And I'm not just talking about at church. I'm talking about at home…at the bank…when you answer the phone and it's a telemarketer… when you are sitting in the stands watching them play ball…or any other public place. Remember: your *way of life* is just that—it's who you are rather than what you do.

Daniel's way of life caused pagan kings to know the one true God. Joseph's way of life allowed him to rise to a place of authority, which then allowed him to save countless lives. Barnabas' way of life earned him the reputation of being an encourager and dedicated leader in the early Church.

A faith worthy to be imitated…do you have that? I've had a few people comment over the years that they don't feel we should be imitating anyone's faith but that of Jesus Christ. While I get what they are saying, scripture clearly indicates that we *are* to set an example and that we *are* supposed to be intertwined with one another in this way.

Elisha so admired Elijah's faith that he asked that it be passed on to him. Elijah, the faithful one, admired the faith of the Widow of Zarephath. Jesus recognized the faith of many; stating that it was their faith that allowed His miraculous powers to heal them.

So where does that leave you?

It leaves you with the task of being the Daniel...the Elijah...the Peter...the Joseph...the best You in the lives of the young people you are associated with. It leaves you with the responsibility to be a person of integrity and spiritual discernment and wisdom. It leaves you with the responsibility to teach, mentor, and live by faith.

Faith...it's what's best for a Great Life.

Chapter 9: Unconditional Love

Of all the things we should want to pass on to the younger people in our lives, unconditional love is the second only to that of desiring to know Christ as their Savior. The knowledge that they are loved unconditionally *as well as* teaching them the importance of importance of loving this way is the foundational cornerstone of living life as the hands, feet, eyes, ears, mouth, and heart of Jesus.

But what is unconditional love?

A friend of mine defines unconditional love as that just because you're you kind of love. It's the kind of love that doesn't depend on what you look like, what you do for a living, how athletic, intellectual, or talented you are.

Unconditional love doesn't notice how much you weigh, how much money is in your bank account, whether or not you have a speech impediment or acne, or anything else.

I've said it before and I'll say it again...passing on this and other Godly character traits is best done when you do them yourself...when you *are* these things, yourself.

Letting the young people in your life know they are loved unconditionally should really be a 'given' for any parent. Sadly, however, it doesn't always work that way. I think we all know someone whose relationship with their parents was performance-based. This simply should not be.

Jesus calls us to love as he loves (John 13:34) and Jesus loves us unconditionally. He didn't just die for the people who believed who he was/is. He didn't just die for the Israelite nation. He didn't just die for those he knew (because of His omnipotence) would someday accept him as Savior. No, Jesus died for *everyone* because He yet loved us even though we were sinners.

You need to understand, though, that unconditional love isn't a 'pass' that gives you the freedom to do whatever you want, whenever you want with total disregard for living a life of faithful obedience to Christ. Jesus loves us unconditionally but His blessings are conditional upon our obedience and faith.

For example, Jesus' love makes salvation available to anyone and everyone, but only those who accept that gift of salvation will be blessed with spending eternity in heaven. Likewise, the unconditional love that led Jesus to the cross is for everyone, but His blessings of comfort in times of grief, provision in times of want, and protection in times of danger are only given to those who are close enough to Him to receive them and recognize that they are from Him.

In the same way we need to let our young people know that there is nothing they can do to lose our love, but that if they want to be blessed in the relationship, they need to hold it in honor. The blessings aren't a condition of our love, but rather a demonstration of our appreciation and joy for the relationship.

I hope this explanation is adequate. I also hope it is a solid reminder that loving unconditionally really isn't an option. It is a command from Jesus according to John 13:34. So as you think about sharing these truths with the young people in your life, remember to do it in such a way that you will reflect the Lord Jesus Christ in a real way.

Chapter 10: Wisdom

As you read these words, consider passing them on to the young people in your life in an effort to help them as they take this journey we call life.

NOTE: Some of the following words of wisdom are original, others are quotes (or variations of) many of you may be familiar with.

Don't ever forget or ignore your children, because they are your life's greatest accomplishment.

If it sounds too good to be true – it probably is.

If you have a Servant's Heart – You won't have a Selfish Heart.

Solitude brings Revelations

Everything is Possible but not Everything is Probable.

Think for Yourself and Learn Directly from God.

Pray for the Best but Prepare for the Worst.

Know Thyself then Be True to Yourself and Live with No Regrets unto God

Don't try to be anyone other than yourself because you aren't equipped to be anyone other than yourself.

Don't ever pass up the opportunity to be kind or bless someone

You get out of life only what you put into it.

When you have a bad day, just remember what a tiny speck that day really is in the big picture of eternity.

No one can make you do anything. Ultimately, you are the only one who can make you do anything.

If you spend your life thinking about what you don't have, you'll never appreciate and enjoy what you do have.

Speak the Truth – Regardless of the Consequences.

God's promises are never broken—we are.

God always has a plan and His plan is always best.

Say what you mean and mean what you say. Always – Let your yes be yes and your no, no.

Don't ever assume you know what someone is thinking or how they feel. Instead, ask them so you'll know for sure and then act accordingly.

Failure isn't a bad thing but accepting it is

God first—always. If you live that way you won't ever have to ask what's next.

God has promised us that in the end, everything will be okay, so if everything isn't okay, you'll know it's not the end.

Remember: Sharing life with the young people in your life isn't just a good idea. It's living life the way God intends.

Special Gift

God has a Gift for You! The Plan of Salvation:

There is no formal prayer of salvation as many churches would have you believe, God's Word is very clear - there is only one way to get to the Father in heaven and that is through Jesus Christ (John 14:6). Jesus says that you must be born again to enter into heaven (John 3:3-5).

Salvation is simply the first step in building an open and honest relationship with God. We all have sinned and fallen short, but there is Hope in Jesus Christ - Just cry out to God in sincerity and honesty asking for forgiveness and for Him to Save you, Sanctify you, and fill you with His Holy Spirit - Ask for His will to be done in your life on earth as it is in Heaven and That's it, now just keep it real with God.

A Warning:

The Christian walk is not an easy life on the surface. The Word of God says that we will be hated in all the world for Christ namesake (Matt. 24:9). The Bible says that in the last days are enemy prevail against us physically until Christ returns to save us (Dan 7:21, 22). Furthermore, we must endure hardship as a good soldier of Jesus Christ (2 Tim 2:3) and yet we are never alone in this, God promises us that He will never leave us nor forsake us if we believe in him (Matt.28:20).

In everything we go through we have the peace and joy of God which surpasses all understanding (Philp. 4:6-8) The Bible declares, "For I consider the sufferings of this present time are not worthy to be compared with the glory which shall be revealed in us". (Rom 8:18). However, in all these things we are more than conquerors through Jesus Christ (Rom. 8:37)

Stay in Contact

Stay in Contact with the American Christian Defense Alliance, Inc. through Our Website At: ACDAInc.Org

Join Our Mailing List

We also Greatly Appreciate You Signing Up For Our Mailing List and Providing a Good Rating and review for this Book. Your reviews help other people like yourself find this book and benefit from its contents.

If You or Your Family have been Blessed by this book please let us know by dropping us a line through our website at ACDAInc.Org

Find All Our Books

Some of Our Books:

Parenting: How To Be A Great Parent And Raise Awesome Kids

Prayer: Your No. 1 Prayer Book To Learn To Be A Strong Christian Prayer Warrior That Prays With Powerful Prayers In The War Room To Overcome And Defeat The Enemy

Salvation for Your Unsaved Mom: 10 Things to Tell Your Mom Before She Dies

Wisdom from Your Elders: Learning From Your Parents, Grandparents, and the Older People in Your Church

Kids and Prayer: Pray with Your Kids and Teach Them How to Pray

Embracing Pregnancy, Your Child, and Parenting: A Christian Parenting Guide to Offer Encouragement During the Wonders, Joy, and Hope of Your First Child

Race Relations in America: A Christian Guide to Unite Christians in the Faith

Martial Arts Ministry: How To Start A Martial Arts Ministry

Biblical Bug Out: Don't Bug In - Follow The Calling

Christian Prepping 101: How To Start Prepping

How to Finance Your Full-Time RV Dream

Make Money: A Beginners Guide to Start an Online Business, Work from Home, Make Money, and Develop Financial Freedom

Additional Formats

Thank you for reading this book. Your support and the support of others continue to humble us and enable our Ministry to grow. We hope and pray that this book has blessed you in some way. If you enjoyed this book consider purchasing it as a gift for someone who could benefit from it.

We Greatly Appreciate Your Support as Well as You Sharing this information, including links to our books with Others on Your Social Media Platforms

Thank You Once Again for Your Support; We Know God Will Bless You as You Have Blessed This Ministry

www.ingramcontent.com/pod-product-compliance
Lightning Source LLC
Chambersburg PA
CBHW021359210526
45463CB00001B/160